LWW's Foundations in
Sterile Products
for Pharmacy Technicians

D1604564

LWW's Foundations in
Sterile Products
for Pharmacy Technicians

W. RENÈE ACOSTA, R.PH, M.S.

University of Texas at Austin,
College of Pharmacy

Wolters Kluwer | Lippincott Williams & Wilkins
Health

Philadelphia · Baltimore · New York · London
Buenos Aires · Hong Kong · Sydney · Tokyo

Acquisitions Editor: David B. Troy
Product Manager: Renee Thomas
Marketing Manager: Shauna Kelley
Design Coordinator: Stephen Druding
Artist: Bot Roda
Manufacturing Coordinator: Margie Orzech
Production Services/Compositor: SPi Technologies

First Edition

© 2011 Lippincott Williams & Wilkins, a Wolters Kluwer business

351 West Camden Street   Two Commerce Square, 2001 Market Street
Baltimore, MD 21201   Philadelphia, PA 19103

Printed in China

Library of Congress Cataloging-in-Publication Data
Acosta, W. Renée.
  LWW's foundations in sterile products for pharmacy technicians / W. Renée Acosta. – 1st ed.
      p. ; cm.
  Other title: Foundations in sterile products for pharmacy technicians
  Includes bibliographical references and index.
  ISBN 978-0-7817-7504-5 (alk. paper)
  1. Drugs–Sterilization. 2. Pharmaceutical technology. I. Lippincott Williams & Wilkins.
  II. Title. III. Title: Foundations in sterile products for pharmacy technicians.
  [DNLM: 1. Sterilization–methods. 2. Technology, Pharmaceutical–standards. 3. Drug Compounding–standards. 4. Drug Contamination–prevention & control. 5. Pharmacists' Aides. QV 778 A185L 2011]
  RS199.S73A36 2011
  615'.19–dc22
                                                          2010014018

DISCLAIMER
Care has been taken to confirm the accuracy of the information present and to describe generally accepted practices. However, the authors, editors, and publisher are not responsible for errors or omissions or for any consequences from application of the information in this book and make no warranty, expressed or implied, with respect to the currency, completeness, or accuracy of the contents of the publication. Application of this information in a particular situation remains the professional responsibility of the practitioner; the clinical treatments described and recommended may not be considered absolute and universal recommendations.

The authors, editors, and publisher have exerted every effort to ensure that drug selection and dosage set forth in this text are in accordance with the current recommendations and practice at the time of publication. However, in view of ongoing research, changes in government regulations, and the constant flow of information relating to drug therapy and drug reactions, the reader is urged to check the package insert for each drug for any change in indications and dosage and for added warnings and precautions. This is particularly important when the recommended agent is a new or infrequently employed drug.

Some drugs and medical devices presented in this publication have Food and Drug Administration (FDA) clearance for limited use in restricted research settings. It is the responsibility of the health care provider to ascertain the FDA status of each drug or device planned for use in their clinical practice.

To purchase additional copies of this book, call our customer service department at **(800) 638-3030** or fax orders to **(301) 223-2320**. International customers should call **(301) 223-2300**.

Visit Lippincott Williams & Wilkins on the Internet: **http://www.lww.com.** Lippincott Williams & Wilkins customer service representatives are available from 8:30 am to 6:00 pm, EST.

                                    9 8 7 6 5 4 3 2 1

Preface

LWW's Foundations in Sterile Products for Pharmacy Technicians is the essential resource on sterile products for pharmacy technician students and their instructors. The most relevant and focused book on the market, it has been developed specifically for pharmacy technician students and programs. Comprehensive yet concise, avoiding fluff or filler, the text is the right depth, the right length, the right choice. Pharmacy technician students who learn their sterile product techniques with this book will be knowledgeable, confident, and prepared for professional success.

LWW's Foundations in Sterile Products for Pharmacy Technicians is organized logically to build knowledge systematically. Students begin by understanding the vital importance of sterile techniques and preparations in the pharmacy and healthcare settings, then move on to contamination prevention and calculations before learning about the role of sterility in equipment and environment. From there, students are ready to understand aseptic techniques, preparation procedures, and finally how to make sterile products. In the text's final chapter, quality assurance procedures are detailed. Throughout the chapters, special features highlight and reinforce key information, while the straightforward writing style engages students and pulls them into the material.

Features

Each chapter of LWW's Foundations in Sterile Products for Pharmacy Technicians includes the following features:

- **Chapter Objectives** prepare the student for each chapter's material by laying out the key topics.
- **Key Terms** set up students' understanding of the material while also providing handy lists for studying at the start of each chapter, including definitions. Terms are bolded and highlighted throughout the chapter for in-context reinforcement.
- **Tips** offer advice for remembering and applying the chapter's content.
- **Proceed with Caution** highlights concepts that have especially high potential for dangerous error.

- **Procedures** provide step-by-step instructions for important skills and tasks.
- **Quick Quizzes** provide in-context self-study and review opportunities for students or assignment options for instructors. Questions are multiple choice, short answer, true-or-false, and matching. Answers are provided in Appendix C.

Chapter 3, Sterile Product Calculations, also includes **Sample Calculations**, which explain in step-by-step detail how to complete pharmaceutical math problems.

Additional Resources

LWW's Foundations in Sterile Products for Pharmacy Technicians includes additional resources for both instructors and students that are available on the book's companion website at http://thePoint.lww.com/AcostaSterileProds.

Approved adopting instructors will be given access to the following additional resources:

- Brownstone Test Generator
- PowerPoint Presentations
- Image Bank
- WebCT and Blackboard Ready Cartridge

Students who have purchased LWW's Foundations in Sterile Products for Pharmacy Technicians have access to:

- An electronic Quiz Bank for independent study and review
- Videos and animations demonstrating sterile techniques as well as drug functions in the body

In addition, instructors and purchasers of the text can access the searchable Full Text On-line by going to the LWW's Foundations in Sterile Products for Pharmacy Technicians website at http://thePoint.lww.com/AcostaSterileProds. See the inside front cover of this text for more details, including the passcode you will need to gain access to the website.

JANET MCGREGOR LILES
Arkansas State University
Beebe, AR

ANITA MOSLEY
University of the Incarnate World
San Antonio, TX

MUGDHA GHOLE
Touro University
Mare Island, CA

MARTA LOPEZ
Miami Dade College-Medical
Miami, FL

DONNA GUISADO
North-West College
West Covina, CA

Contents

CHAPTER 1

Sterile Product Basics

CHAPTER OBJECTIVES

- Describe the importance of sterility and how to validate the sterility of a product.
- List the different routes of administration for compounded sterile products.
- Compare and contrast the importance of sterility when compounding medications for the various routes of administration.
- Describe the advantages and disadvantages of the different routes of parenteral administration.
- Outline the history of sterile product guidelines and laws.
- Identify the advantages of having pharmacy personnel compound sterile products.
- Differentiate the roles of the pharmacy technician and the pharmacist in the preparation of sterile products.

KEY TERMS

autoclave—a machine invented in 1879 to sterilize equipment and other objects using superheated water and pressurized steam

biologic indicator—a special preparation of microorganisms that are known to be resistant to a particular sterilization process

catheter—a delivery or drainage tube that is inserted into a vein, artery, or body cavity

compounded sterile product (CSP)—a mixture of one or more substances that is made free of contamination before use

continuous infusion—when a volume of 250 mL or more is injected into a vein and administered at a constant flow rate

intermittent infusion—when a volume of 500 mL or less is given over a shorter time period than a continuous infusion and combined with other fluids

intravenous (IV) admixture—a CSP in which a measured substance is added to a 50 mL or larger bag or bottle of IV fluid

intravenous push (IVP)—a method of drug administration in which a small volume of medicine (less than 250 mL) is injected into a vein and administered over a short period of time

ophthalmics—drugs applied to the eye

otics—drugs applied to the ear

parenteral—a compound that is given by injection

pyrogens—fever-producing organic substances such as bacteria, viruses, or fungi

route of administration—the specific way a parenteral or other drug comes into contact with body tissue

sterilization—the destruction of all living organisms and their spores from a preparation

---

In the past, traditional pharmacists were required to compound anything the physician ordered. Today, as a pharmacy technician, you may encounter many medications that will already come prepared from the manufacturer. However, there's a wide range of products that simply can't be prepared ahead of time or outside of a sterile setting. This requires that pharmacy staff understand the processes of sterile compounding to prepare these orders.

In this chapter, you'll learn the basics of preparing **compounded sterile products (CSPs)**, such as the importance of sterility, the primary methods of sterilization, and how to validate the sterility of a CSP. You will learn about different routes of administration, such as parenterals, including the intravenous (IV), intradermal (ID), intramuscular (IM), and subcutaneous routes.

It is important for you as a pharmacy technician to know the history of sterility. You will learn when the first technology for preparing sterile products was developed and when laws requiring sterile procedures were first established. Finally, you'll learn about the advantages of having pharmacy staff prepare sterile products in a controlled environment.

THE IMPORTANCE OF STERILITY

One of your most important tasks as a pharmacy technician is preparing compounded sterile products, or CSPs. A CSP is a mixture of one or more substances that is made sterile, or free of contamination, before use. As you might guess, a CSP must be sterile before it comes into contact with living tissue. If the product is contaminated, the results could be lethal.

You do your job toward guaranteeing this by preparing CSPs in only the cleanest, most controlled conditions. This may sound difficult, but it's a little easier than it sounds. Well-established guidelines already exist that describe how to prepare CSPs under controlled conditions. You simply need to make sure you follow these guidelines and know how to use the resources put in place for sterile compounding. This will ensure that you are practicing the most effective technique possible.

Pyrogens

The main reason for practicing good sterile technique is to prevent particles or **pyrogens**—fever-producing organic substances such as bacteria, viruses, or fungi—from mixing with a CSP. A fever that develops after administering an intravenous (IV) drug is usually the result of pyrogen contamination. Keeping pyrogens from contaminating a CSP is one of your most critical challenges as a pharmacy technician.

Basic Product Sterility

The term **sterilization** refers to the destruction of all living organisms and their spores from a preparation. There are five basic methods used to sterilize pharmaceutical products:

- steam
- dry heat
- filtration
- gas
- ionizing radiation

The method is determined largely by the nature of the preparation and its ingredients. You'll learn more about these methods in Chapter 9.

Validation of Sterility

How do you know if a CSP is free of contamination? As precise as your technique and sterilization methods may be, CSPs must still be validated to make sure they are free from contamination. Validation includes testing, visually inspecting, and closely reviewing CSPs to assure that the finished product meets purity and quality standards.

The Biologic Indicator

One way to make sure a CSP is sterile is to use a **biologic indicator**—a special preparation of harmless microorganisms that are known to be resistant to a particular sterilization process. The biologic indicator is almost always used to test the validity in high-risk-level CSPs. Here's how it works:

1. Spores of the indicator are added to a product before sterilization.
2. The product is sterilized using the appropriate method for that specific CSP.
3. The product is examined to see if the spores survived.
4. If the spores have been killed, this indicates that sterilization was successful.

Visual Inspection

Once the CSPs have been prepared, it's time to inspect and label the products. At this time, you must visually inspect the CSPs. Visual inspection of a product is as simple as comparing the actual appearance to the expected appearance, including the final fill amount.

How do you know what the CSP should look like? The supplier may provide literature describing the expected appearance, which should be stored in the lab and readily accessible.

Visual inspection includes squeezing the bag to make sure you did not accidentally puncture it during preparation. It also involves holding the product against a light background and a dark background to make sure there are no particles floating in the bag. These particles may be particulate matter caused by poor technique or a precipitate which results when drugs are not compatible together. The ability to visually inspect a CSP is something that pharmacy technicians gain with experience and practice.

CSP Review

Visually inspecting a CSP will help you determine if there is particulate matter. But you must also verify its concentration, strength, and purity. This verification process is completed by reviewing the following:

- labels on packages
- certificates of analysis provided by suppliers
- other approved processes or devices for verification set in place by individual labs

ROUTES OF ADMINISTRATION

The specific way a drug comes into contact with body tissue is its **route of administration**. Usually the physician, physician's assistant, or nurse is responsible for administering a drug. But still, it's important for you as a pharmacy technician to understand the process of administration. Occasionally, a patient may ask a question about a drug he has received. But more importantly, the specific ways in which you prepare certain drugs often depend on the route of administration.

You'll learn much more about preparing sterile products in future chapters. But for now, let's take a look at some of the common routes of administration.

Parenterals

The majority of sterile products a pharmacy technician will compound are called parenterals. **Parenterals** are medications that are injected. Why do you think it is so important that parenterals be sterile?

A parenteral may be injected under the skin or into a joint, the spinal column, a muscle, a vein, an artery, or even the heart. Parenterals are absorbed quickly in areas where the body's defense mechanisms do not have a chance to work. If pyrogens are administered directly into the body, death or major complications such as phlebitis (inflammation of a vein) or sepsis (the presence of organisms in the blood) could occur.

Here are some situations that would call for a parenteral route of administration:

- when a medication cannot be taken by mouth or other non-invasive route (e.g., nasal)
- when a rapid response is desired
- when the patient is unconscious
- when a medication would be ineffective using other routes

Here are a few routes used in the medical setting on a high-frequency basis:

- intravenous
- subcutaneous
- intramuscular
- intradermal

Intravenous (IV) Injections

An intravenous (IV) injection is one that goes directly into a vein. The type of CSP injected is called an **intravenous (IV) admixture**—a measured substance added to a 50 mL or larger bag or bottle of IV fluid. An intravenous injection is the most common parenteral route of administration.

IV injection is the fastest parenteral route of administration. Since drug absorption is not a factor, optimum blood levels may be achieved with accuracy

PROCEED WITH CAUTION

Disadvantages of IV Injections

On the negative side of IVs, once a drug is administered intravenously, it cannot be retrieved. The drug cannot easily be removed from the body, as it could, for example, by induction of vomiting after oral administration of the same drug.

Also, the possibility of particulate matter in IV solutions is a constant concern. Therefore, great care must be taken to prepare sterile, accurate dosing of IV solutions.

and immediacy not possible by other routes. In emergencies, IV administration of a drug may be lifesaving because the drug is placed directly into the circulation.

T I P Any volume of medicine can be delivered using IV administration. This is a distinct advantage over other methods, which have a limit on the volume of medicine that can be administered in one site. It's convenient for alternative and split dosing as well.

An IV injection can be given one of two ways:

- intravenous push (IVP)
- intravenous infusion

Intravenous Push (IVP) and Intravenous Infusion

An **intravenous push** is a small volume of medicine that is injected into a vein and administered over a short period of time.

For intravenous infusion, a needle is placed in a prominent vein of the forearm or leg and taped firmly to the patient so that it will not slip from place during infusion. An IV fluid and the drug is administered either continuously or intermittently.

- Continuous Infusion—a patient receives a **continuous infusion** when a volume of 250 mL or more is injected into a vein or catheter and administered at a constant flow rate.
- Intermittent Infusion—a patient receives an **intermittent infusion** when a volume of 500 mL or less is given over a shorter time period. This dilutes the IV medicine, making it less irritating to the vein.

Catheter Lines

When parenteral administration has to be repeated over time, it makes more sense to use a catheter. A **catheter** is a delivery or drainage tube that is inserted into a vein, artery, or body cavity (Fig. 1-1). Fluids can be drained or injected using a catheter line.

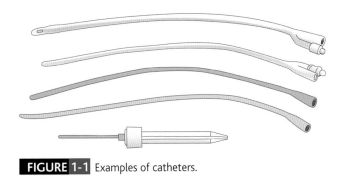

FIGURE 1-1 Examples of catheters.

Catheters make repeated parenteral administration much easier since they eliminate the need for multiple punctures. Using a single catheter puncture also makes it easier to reduce the risk of contamination.

There are two basic types of venous catheter lines:

- central venous line
- peripheral venous line

Central Venous Catheter Line

A central venous catheter line is one that is placed into a large vein in the neck, chest, or groin. This type of venous catheter can stay in place for a few days to several months. It can be used for a variety of parenteral medicines, including the following:

- cancer chemotherapy
- long-term antibiotic therapy
- total parenteral nutrition solutions

Sterile technique is very important when using any type of catheter line. A catheter line could easily serve as a place of entry for pyrogens or other contaminating substances. Or the catheter line itself may become infected. Therefore, the care of catheter lines is critically important.

Peripheral Catheter Line

A peripheral catheter line is one that is inserted in either the arms or the hands. Medicines or solutions are then injected into the peripheral line. Since these lines are the easiest to put in place, they are the most frequent routes of IV administration.

Subcutaneous

Some parenterals do not need to be delivered directly into the vein. A subcutaneous injection places the drug into the tissues between the skin and the muscle. A subcutaneous injection is slower acting than an intramuscular injection.

Patients who inject themselves with insulin use this type of parenteral route. Only volumes up to 2.0 mL can be injected this way. As is the case with any parenteral, the injection site should always be thoroughly cleaned with antibacterial cleanser to prevent infection.

Intramuscular (IM)

Some parenterals may be delivered more deeply than a subcutaneous injection. An intramuscular (IM) injection is quicker acting than a subcutaneous injection. The effects are slower in onset than IV, but will last longer.

The injection is delivered deep within the buttock, thigh, or upper arm muscle. The biggest drawback to an IM injection is the pain that usually results from it. In addition, there are maximum volumes that can be administered at one time in one site: for adults, a total of 5 mL; for children, a total of 2 mL; for neonates, a total of 0.5 mL. If more volume is needed, then the volume should be split into two syringes and administered at two different sites.

Intradermal (ID)

Very small amounts of medicine (about 0.1 mL) are sometimes injected using an intradermal (ID) route. This parenteral route delivers the medicine below the upper layer of skin, into the vascular (containing blood vessels) layer. The front of the forearm is often the site for this type of injection.

Other Injectables

Again, IV, subcutaneous, IM, and ID are the most common routes of parenteral administration. There are a few others that you should be familiar with even though they are not used as frequently. These injections include the following:

- intra-articular—administered into the articular cartilage of a joint
- intrasynovial—administered into the joint fluid area
- intraspinal—administered into the spinal column
- intrathecal—administered into the spinal fluid
- intra-arterial—administered into an artery
- intracardiac—administered into the heart

 PROCEED WITH CAUTION

Coat the Catheter

The use of a central venous catheter line carries the risk of contamination and infection of the bloodstream. If the catheter is scheduled to be in place for more than five days, physicians recommend that a coated catheter be used. Such catheter lines are coated both internally and externally with antiseptics or antibiotics.

TIP Always remember the importance of good sterile technique. As a pharmacy technician, you must take every precaution necessary to avoid contamination. The parenteral route is the most dangerous route of administration because it bypasses all of the body's natural defenses. An improperly prepared parenteral, when administered, can lead to infections, emboli, occlusions, and even death.

Other Dosage Forms

Most dosage forms that are not injected are administered where the body's natural defenses can filter or destroy unwanted substances. By developing familiarity with these compounds, you can gain a better understanding of which products require complete sterile preparation and which do not.

Most of these products require that steps be taken for preservation to avoid microbial growth. But, with the exception of ophthalmics, they do not require the high levels of precaution and control as sterile products administered by the parenteral route. Some of these products are ophthalmics, enterals, nasal preparations, and otics.

Ophthalmics

Ophthalmics are drugs applied topically to the eye and are prepared as gels, solutions, and ointments. They are used to treat surface or intraocular conditions such as the following:

- bacterial, fungal, and viral infections
- allergic reactions
- inflammation
- glaucoma
- dryness

Unlike other body parts, such as the nose and ear, the eye is composed of highly sensitive tissue with no outer layer of defense. Any pyrogens or particle matter in a medication will be absorbed, thus contaminating the eye and causing irritation, a scratched cornea, or both.

Enterals

Enterals are products that are taken orally, or through the mouth. These include tablets, capsules, elixirs, syrups, solutions, oral suspensions, and lozenges.

Most enterals are absorbed in the intestines and must pass through the stomach, which produces hydrochloric acid (HCl). Hydrochloric acid has a pH of about 2. You'll learn more about pH in Chapter 2, but most pyrogens cannot survive under such conditions. Therefore, enterals do not need to be prepared as sterile products.

PROCEED WITH CAUTION

Ear Trauma

Patients should be thoroughly examined before otics are prescribed. If there is broken skin in the ear canal, or the ear drum is punctured, certain ingredients in some otics, such as boric acid, may be toxic.

Nasal Preparations

Most nasal preparations are intended for intranasal use and produce a local effect. The majority of these are in solution form and are administered as nose drops, sprays, and, sometimes, jellies. Nasal preparations must be stabilized and preserved to avoid antimicrobial contamination.

Otics

Otics are drugs in drop or ointment form that are administered into the ear. These products are usually administered to the ear canal in small amounts. They are used to treat the following:

- excess earwax
- ear infections
- inflammation or pain

Since otics are administered to the ear canal, which is covered by layers of skin, high-risk preparation is not required. Like nasal compounds, some liquid otic preparations require preservation against microbial growth.

A STERILE CHALLENGE

People have been compounding medicines for thousands of years. However, the challenge of keeping tools and medicines free of contamination has been approached in various ways.

One of the first methods was to use fire to heat tools to a red-hot glow. Although fire, a dry heat, could be helpful in sterilizing certain metal tools, it could not be used for medicines, plastics, or other nonmetal items.

Scientists and physicians have gradually refined their sterile practices over time.

Autoclave

The technology for producing sterile products probably began in 1679 with French chemist Denis Papin's invention of the pressure cooker. This locked, sealed metal pot is still used today. It uses superheated steam to cook food quickly without destroying valuable nutrients.

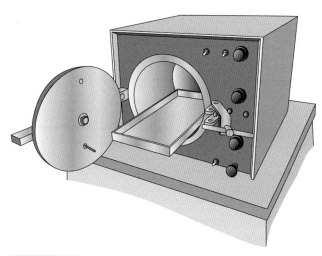

FIGURE 1-2 The autoclave uses steam to kill bacteria, fungi, spores, and viruses on medical equipment.

The pressure cooker was the forerunner to the **autoclave**, a machine invented in 1879 that uses moist heat in the form of steam to sterilize equipment and other objects. The autoclaves of today are available in various sizes and are used extensively in the medical environment (Fig. 1-2).

MODERN STERILE PRACTICES

The importance of practicing efficient sterile preparation in the pharmacy was not seriously addressed until the 1960s and 1970s. Sterility became a critical issue at this time after many patient deaths and injuries due to contaminated compounding and administration.

The National Coordinating Committee on Large Volume Parenterals (NCCLVP)

The NCCLVP was officially one of the first organizations to attempt to set standard guidelines of practice for CSPs. Its recommendations addressed preparation, labeling, and quality assurance of CSPs for hospitals.

Unfortunately the organization was dissolved shortly after its recommendations were launched. This again left pharmacies and hospitals with no set standards or reinforcement.

Sterile Organizations Combine

After the disbanding of the NCCLVP, several organizations were forced to step in to provide some sort of structure to sterile compounding. These included the following:

- American Society of Health-System Pharmacists (ASHP)
- United States Pharmacopeia (USP)
- National Association of Boards of Pharmacy (NABP)

Throughout the 1980s and 1990s, these organizations issued various combinations of recommendations and guidelines in regard to labeling, preparing, storing, dispensing, and administering CSPs. But ultimately, no official, universal regulations existed.

USP Chapter 797

On January 1, 2004, USP Chapter 797 of the United States Pharmacopeia and the National Formulary (USP) was published as the first official and enforceable document to outline set standards for CSPs.

The USP Chapter 797 requirements are incorporated into the sterile technique followed by all pharmacists and pharmacy technicians. These guidelines help to ensure the proper preparation, labeling, storage, and administration of compound sterile products.

A Bit of History

As you have learned, it took a while for the USP to initiate such a long-overdue doctrine. Still, it makes sense that the USP would be the organization to do so, considering its extensive history. Let's take a quick look:

- 1906—Congress and the USP pass the Food and Drugs Act
- 1938—Congress passes the Federal Food, Drug, and Cosmetic (FD&C) Act (a revision of the 1906 act)
- 1938—The FD&C appoints the USP the official compendia of drug standards

Sterile Enforcement

USP Chapter 797 is considered a requirement. As a requirement, those standards and guidelines may be inspected by a number of organizations, including the following:

- U.S. Boards of Pharmacy
- U.S. Food and Drug Administration
- The Joint Commission
- Accreditation Commission for Health Care, Inc. (ACHC)
- Community Health Accreditation Program (CHAP)

State of Practice

Each state has a separate board of pharmacy that may enforce activities differently. Therefore, in addition to closely following the guidelines set in USP Chapter 797, pharmacists should contact their state board for specific regulations.

CSP Flexibility

The USP recognized that the facilities in which sterile products are prepared are vastly different. To accommodate such discrepancies, the USP wrote Chapter 797 to give pharmacists a bit of flexibility. Ultimately, it is the pharmacist who is responsible for determining the different levels of risk, and necessary precautions, for compounding each sterile compound. You will learn more about specific risk factors in the chapters to come.

ADVANTAGES OF PHARMACY-PREPARED STERILE PRODUCTS

There are many advantages to pharmacy-prepared sterile products:

- highly skilled professionals who know the drugs and know the processes
- quality assurance systems
- controlled environment in which sterile resources are put to use

Without the advantages of professionally prepared sterile products, the risk of contamination is high and the patient's life is in jeopardy.

Trained Personnel

The current regulations and guidelines require that all pharmacy technicians go through extensive training in sterile compound preparation. This is accomplished both by learning and by practicing the steps of proper aseptic technique. In addition, both pharmacists and technicians are evaluated and assessed on a regular basis. You'll learn more about this in Chapter 9.

Double Checks

In the past, a CSP would have been prepared and no steps would have been taken to double-check the accuracy or quality of the product. Today, the work of pharmacy technicians is routinely double-checked by pharmacists.

A Clean, Controlled Environment

Before the widespread knowledge of the risks of contamination, many medicines were compounded and prepared in a patient's room. Such conditions were certainly not sterile.

Today, the environment in which products are prepared is controlled and maintained to specific levels of cleanliness. One of the largest improvements in the preparation of CSPs is the enforcement of a designated space for preparation. This makes much more efficient use of all resources. In other words, there is one place for CSP preparation, not several places used on an on-demand basis.

Every controlled environment is required to meet the USP Chapter 797 guidelines. Here are some environmental and resource requirements:

- A laminar-airflow workbench, clean room, and barrier isolator all must be maintained and certified regularly.
- The compounding area is separate from the general pharmacy and has a controlled (particle, temperature, and humidity) environment.
- A clean environment is maintained for areas where CSPs are exposed to the physical environment.
- Detailed cleaning and sanitizing procedures are followed to maintain the cleanliness of the compounding environment.
- Personnel are always properly garbed.
- The compounding environment is routinely monitored.

You will learn much more about these resources in future chapters.

CHAPTER HIGHLIGHTS

- Dosage forms whose routes of administration bypass the body's natural defenses must be sterile. This is especially true of parenterals.
- The validation of CSPs includes testing, visual inspection, and close review.
- The specific way a drug comes into contact with body tissue is its route of administration.
- The most frequently used routes of parenteral administration are intravenous, intramuscular, subcutaneous, and intradermal.
- Smaller volumes are injected using the subcutaneous and intradermal routes of administration. The intramuscular route of administration is usually the most painful.
- A central venous catheter line is one that is placed into a large vein in the neck, chest, or groin. A peripheral catheter line is one that is inserted in either the arms or the hands.
- Strict regulations and guidelines regarding the procedures and requirements for compounding CSPs were first published in USP Chapter 797 of the United States Pharmacopeia (USP) and the National Formulary (N.F.) in 2004. Before that time, no official, enforceable regulations existed.
- The advantages of having CSPs prepared by pharmacy personnel include the assurance that current guidelines and regulations are followed.
- The pharmacy technician is responsible for following all necessary requirements in preparing, compounding, and packaging CSPs. The pharmacist is responsible for double-checking that the pharmacy technician follows all current regulations and guidelines.

QUICK QUIZ

Answer the following multiple-choice questions.

1. All of the following are processes important to CSP validation EXCEPT:
   a. visual inspection.
   b. testing using a biologic indicator.
   c. storing the product for one week to observe changes.
   d. reviewing information provided by suppliers.
2. Which group of CSPs must be sterile?
   a. otics
   b. parenterals
   c. inhalants
   d. enterals
3. All of the following is true of intravenous injections EXCEPT that:
   a. they are convenient for alternative dosing.
   b. optimum levels of a drug can be achieved with high accuracy.
   c. they are the most common parenteral route of administration.
   d. they are not as fast as the oral route of administration.
4. Which statement about ophthalmics is true?
   a. Ophthalmics must be prepared as sterile products.
   b. An ophthalmic is a type of parenteral.
   c. Ophthalmics are used in the ears and do not require sterile preparation.
   d. Ophthalmics are manufactured as drops, ointments, and injections.
5. In what year did the first official regulations for CSPs become enforceable?
   a. 1964
   b. 1974
   c. 1994
   d. 2004

Please answer each of the following questions in a few sentences.

1. Explain why certain compounds that pharmacy technicians are responsible for preparing do not need to be compounded as sterile products in a controlled environment. Provide two examples of these compounds and explain why they do not require as much control as sterile compounds such as parenterals.

_____

_____

2. Explain the difference between a central catheter line and a peripheral catheter line.

_____

_____

3. Name the four most common parenteral routes of administration and explain where in the body they are injected.

_____

_____

4. Describe the two types of IV injections.

_____

_____

5. Discuss two ways that help ensure that sterile conditions for preparing CSPs are maintained.

_____

_____

Answer the following statements as either true or false.

1. ____ An IV push would most likely be used to administer 225 mL of medicine over a 48-hour period.
2. ____ The parenteral route is the most dangerous route of administration.
3. ____ The autoclave uses dry heat, such as a flame, to sterilize medical equipment.
4. ____ The FDA published Chapter 797, the first comprehensive and enforceable set of guidelines for sterile product preparation.
5. ____ Each pharmacist must follow strict guidelines in determining the risk factor for sterile products regardless of facility resources or location.

Match the term in the left column with the correct description from the right column.

1. pyrogen
2. biologic indicator
3. parenteral
4. route of administration
5. catheter

a. the specific way a parenteral or other drug comes into contact with body tissue
b. a delivery or drainage tube that is inserted into a vein, artery, or body cavity
c. fever-producing organic substances such as bacteria, viruses, or fungi
d. a CSP that is given by injection
e. a special preparation of microorganisms that are known to be resistant to a particular sterilization process

CHAPTER 2

Preventing Contamination

- Identify different ways that CSPs can become contaminated.
- Define touch contamination.
- Describe shadowing.
- Describe ways to minimize microbial contamination when compounding CSPs.
- Define stability.
- Explain storage conditions commonly required for CSPs.
- Define the beyond-use date of a CSP.
- Differentiate between the expiration date and the beyond-use date of a CSP.
- Define compatibility and incompatibility.
- Identify different types of incompatibility.
- Describe how the pH affects the stability and compatibility of CSPs.
- Define the terms isotonic, hypertonic, and hypotonic.
- Describe the effects on the body of intravenous hypertonic versus hypotonic CSPs.
- Define osmotic pressure.
- Explain the importance of osmolality and osmolarity of CSPs.

KEY **TERMS**

absorption—the process that occurs when an ingredient is soaked up by the CSP container and results in loss of drug

adsorption—the process that occurs when an ingredient adheres to the surface of the CSP container and results in loss of drug

beyond-use date—the date after which a product must not be used; determined by the pharmacist from the date and time the product is prepared

buffer—a compound or mixture of compounds that helps prevent changes in pH

compatibility—a property that describes how effectively one product will combine with another product

contaminant—any unwanted particulate matter or fever-inducing agent

critical area—an ISO Class 5 environment in which CSPs are prepared (e.g., laminar airflow workbench, biological safety cabinet)

critical site—any location where contaminants might come into contact with a CSP; these locations are either never touched (e.g., needle, needle hub, syringe plunger) or swabbed with alcohol prior to needle entry (e.g., ampule, vial stopper)

expiration date—the date after which a product must not be used; determined by the manufacturer for an unopened and properly stored product

incompatibility—a property that describes the negative effect of combining one sterile product with another sterile product, surface, or material

microbial contamination—a situation in which microbes such as bacteria, viruses, molds, or yeasts, come into contact with a CSP

osmolality—the number of osmoles of solute per kilogram of solvent (mOsm/kg)

osmolarity—the number of osmoles of solute per liter of solution (mOsm/L)

pH—the measurement of a substance describing how acidic or basic it is

precipitate—a solid formed from a solution or suspension when incompatible ingredients are combined

shadowing—a situation in which the HEPA-filtered airflow in the critical area (BSC) is blocked before reaching the critical site

stability—the ability of the CSP to remain effective until used, or until the expiration date or beyond-use date has been reached

storage—the area where the CSPs are stored and the container in which each CSP is stored

tonicity—a measurement of the way cells and tissues react to a solution that surrounds them

touch contamination—a situation that occurs when physical contact between a CSP and another object results in contamination; this is the most common cause of contamination when preparing CSPs

---

As a pharmacy technician, one of your primary tasks will be to prepare compounded sterile products (CSPs). When preparing CSPs, you must take great care and effort to maintain sterility.

In this chapter, you'll learn about the critical sites of contamination, how to keep unwanted particles and microbes from contacting CSPs, and how to safely store CSPs. You'll also learn about some properties of CSPs such as stability, dating systems, compatibility, buffers and pH, tonicity, osmolality, and osmolarity.

CONTAMINANTS

As a CSP is prepared, it is important that it remain sterile, or free from **contaminants**. A contaminant is any unwanted particulate matter or fever-inducing agent.

Fibers from clothing or other objects, dust, glass, plastic, metals, bacteria, molds, fungi, and viruses are all examples of contaminants. If one or more of these substances comes into contact with a sterile CSP, the CSP becomes contaminated. There are two ways that CSPs can become contaminated:

- physical contamination (touch contamination, shadowing)
- microbial contamination

As a pharmacy technician, you need to know how contaminants find their way into CSPs. You must also learn ways to prevent CSP contamination.

Physical Contamination

Physical contamination can happen when objects touch each other. It can also happen when contaminated air touches objects in a laminar airflow workbench or biological safety cabinet.

Touch Contamination

The most likely way for CSP contamination to occur is by **touch contamination**. This happens when physical contact between a CSP and another object results in contamination. Any time you handle a CSP, there is a risk of touch contamination. Tiny fibers are constantly shed from your clothes, your hair, and your skin.

From the moment a CSP is prepared to the point it is delivered, time and effort must be taken to prevent touch contamination. This is why wearing protective clothing, wearing gloves, and correct hand washing is especially important. Careful hand washing removes nearly all of the microbes commonly found on the hands: *Staphylococcus*, *Corynebacteria*, and yeasts. Wearing protective clothing and garb that covers the hair and mouth and does not shed fibers lowers the risk of touch contamination.

Critical Site

The **critical site** is any location where contaminants might come into contact with a CSP. This could be any opening or surface at which CSPs and contaminants can meet. Remember that CSPs can also come in contact with contaminants from the air. Some critical sites are exposed to the air and any contaminants in it. These include the:

- tip of a sterile syringe (Fig. 2-1)
- opened ampule of a drug
- injection port

We will discuss critical sites in more detail in Chapter 4.

Another critical site is any mucosal surface of the body. For this reason, isopropyl alcohol (IPA) is often used to clean, or swab, the injection site on the body just before injection.

Time and surface area are important, too. The larger the critical site and the longer it is exposed, the greater the risk of contamination.

! PROCEED WITH CAUTION

Counter Contamination Checklist

Here is a checklist to help you make sure touch contamination never happens:

- Avoid wearing any makeup or jewelry when working in the clean room.
- Always thoroughly scrub hands and arms to the elbow.
- After scrubbing, put on (in order) non-shedding garb including hair covers, face mask, shoe covers, coats or coveralls, and gloves.
- Sanitize all equipment, containers, and surfaces.
- Avoid touching any part of a container or surface that comes into contact with a CSP.

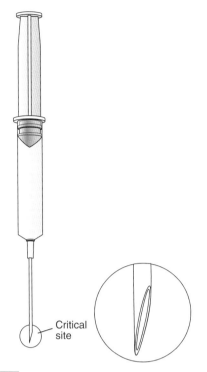

Critical
site

FIGURE 2-1 The tip of a needle is an example of a critical site.

Critical Area

The terms *critical site* and *critical area* sound similar and mean similar things. You already know what a critical site is. A critical area is a place where CSPs, containers, and closures are exposed to the environment. This is where sterile products can be safely prepared or compounded while keeping the risk of contamination very low.

In an ISO Class 5 environment, the critical area has no more than 3,520 particles per cubic meter of air. Laminar airflow workbenches, biological safety cabinets (BSCs), and compounding aseptic isolators are examples of ISO Class 5 environments.

Shadowing

When preparing CSPs in a laminar airflow workbench (LAFW), the air is blowing in a straight line from the HEPA filter out towards you. For this reason, the placement of objects on the work surface is very important. The HEPA filtered air should touch all critical sites and not be blocked.

When preparing CSPs that contain hazardous ingredients, the air right around the product can be quite toxic. For this reason, you and other pharmacy technicians will use a biological safety cabinet, or BSC, for preparing CSPs. In a BSC, the HEPA filtered air is blowing in a straight line from the top to the work surface. The air and fumes are then circulated away from the technician and into a vent.

If the airflow in the LAFW or BSC is blocked, a situation known as **shadowing** occurs. The first air that

touches the CSP should always be the HEPA filtered area. If you are shadowing while preparing your CSP, then the chance of contamination increases. To prevent shadowing, you should always be aware of where you place materials in the hood and where your hands are during product manipulation.

Area of Turbulence

Remember that in most "hooded" work areas, the HEPA (filtered) air is moving horizontally. This means the air is being blown toward you in a straight line. A hooded area with no objects inside contains only HEPA filtered air. So what happens once you introduce an object into the hood? As part of your job, you will need to move objects like IV bags and bottles and vials, and even your own hands, into the hood. This creates an area where HEPA air mixes with unfiltered room air.

Consider this example. When you set a vial inside a laminar hood, filtered air moves toward the vial in a straight line. When this air reaches the vial, it has to move around it. This creates a triangular-shaped area behind the vial. In this area is a mixture of HEPA air and unfiltered room air. This area is also referred to as the *area of turbulence*.

As the vial increases in size, so does the area of turbulence. Always place objects in a straight line when setting them inside a the hood. Never place them in front or back of each other.

Microbial Contamination

The second way that CSPs can become contaminated is through **microbial contamination**. This happens when microbes come into contact with a CSP. These harmful microbes include:

- bacteria
- viruses
- molds
- yeasts

You cannot see microbes without the use of a microscope, but they are everywhere. You can find microbes:

- in the air
- on countertops
- on hands and arms
- in hair
- on clothing

The most likely microbes found in CSPs are those shed by humans. Proper hand scrubbing with antimicrobial cleanser, wearing gloves, hair covers, face masks, and low-particulate clothing are necessary when preparing CSPs.

Of course, eating, drinking, chewing gum and smoking are prohibited in the clean room. All makeup and jewelry must be removed prior to entering the clean room. Even talking is best kept to a minimum. When you talk, airborne particles and microbes move through the air. This increases the risk of contamination.

STERILE PRODUCT PROPERTIES

As a pharmacy technician, you will spend a lot of time preparing CSPs. So it's important to understand the properties of CSPs. This section will describe several properties of sterile products, including:

- stability
- storage
- dating
- pH levels
- compatibility
- tonicity
- osmolality
- osmolarity

Stability

The **stability** of a CSP is its ability to remain effective until used, or until the expiration date or beyond use date has been reached (more on the expiration date and beyond use date later in the chapter). A loss of stability affects the properties and/or effectiveness of a product.

There are several factors that affect a CSP's stability. These include:

- light sensitivity
- chemical reactions
- temperature
- length of time on shelf before use

Storage

Storing CSPs properly helps guarantee their stability. The **storage** of a CSP means not only the area where the CSPs are stored, but the container in which each product is stored.

Approved storage areas for CSPs include designated refrigerators, freezers, or locked cabinets. The type of container storing a CSP is also important.

Recommended Storage Conditions

The United States Pharmacopeia (USP) recommends that CSPs be stored as directed on the label of the ingredients in the CSP. The USP also advises that CSPs be discarded under the following conditions:

- The CSP has been exposed to temperatures higher than the warm limit on the label.
- The CSP has been exposed to temperatures above 40 degrees Celsius for more than four hours.

Storage Monitoring

The USP recommends that CSP storage areas be inspected and checked regularly. This helps ensure that temperature, light, moisture, and airflow are adequately balanced. One of your tasks as a pharmacy technician may include the monitoring of CSP storage areas. Also, remember that all storage areas must be kept as free from contamination as possible. The less traffic in and out of a storage area, the better!

Beyond-Use Dating

All CSPs should have a beyond-use date on the container. This is often confused with the expiration date of a product. Here's an easy way to remember the difference between the two:

- **Expiration date**—placed on the label of a product by the *manufacturer*.
- **Beyond-use date**—placed on the IV label that is affixed to the CSP container and is determined by the *pharmacist*.

The beyond-use date is the date after which a product must not be stored or transported. It is determined by the pharmacist and is based on the following factors:

- the manufacturer's expiration date of each ingredient in the CSP
- the nature of the final CSP
- the characteristics and properties of the container
- expected storage conditions for the product during the time of use

Usually the beyond-use date of the entire CSP is shorter than the expiration date of any single ingredient making up the CSP. Keep in mind that improper storage and/or handling of any CSP will affect the beyond-use date.

Sources of Information

The pharmacist will use different sources of information to determine a CSPs beyond-use date. Information about a CSP's beyond-use date can be found on the package insert that comes with the CSP. These are usually written in an easy-to-read style and include information about when not to use the CSP, how and with what solution to reconstitute a powder, and what base solutions can be used for dilution. Since the package insert is the most accurate information for the product being used, it should be the first source used.

If the package insert does not have sufficient information, several other sources are available. More information can be found in the *Handbook on Injectable*

Drugs (Trissel), The King Guide to Parenteral Admixtures, and *Extended Stability for Parenteral Drugs (Bing).* If the information is not found in any of these sources, the pharmacist may need to look in primary literature to see if any recently published studies have been done. Of course, the pharmacist must use their professional judgment when information is conflicting or not available.

Compatibility

The property of **compatibility** describes how effectively one product will combine with another product. As a pharmacy technician, you will combine and compound many products. The compatibility of different sterile products is extremely important. Not all sterile products combine readily with one another. When incompatible products combine, a physical and/or chemical change may result. These changes may impact the effectiveness and potency of the products.

Incompatibility

The property of **incompatibility** describes the negative effects of combining one sterile product with another sterile product, surface, or material. When incompatible products are combined, a precipitate or gas may be produced; the potency of a product might be reduced. Or, the action of one product may cancel the action of the other product. The property of incompatibility can be categorized as either physical incompatibility or chemical incompatibility.

Physical Incompatibility

Physical incompatibility is the easier kind of incompatibility to identify. When there is a physical incompatibility between two sterile products, a physical change, a change you can usually see or feel, occurs. These changes include:

- cloudiness
- an increase or decrease in cold temperature produced while mixing
- a change in color
- separation

Solubility

Solubility occurs when a *solute* does not dissolve in a *solvent*; one result of incompatibility due to solubility is the formation of a precipitate. This is solid matter that forms when a solute and a solvent are mixed together. For example, in parenteral nutrition mixtures (IV feeding), calcium and phosphate must be mixed together in precise proportions. If they are not, a solid **precipitate**, (a solid formed from a solution or suspension) forms that then blocks the flow of the mixture.

Other solubility issues that you may encounter:

- When adding a drug to an IV bag, the drug must be soluble in the base solution. For example, phenytoin is not soluble in Dextrose 5% in water or Normal saline, which are two commonly used base solutions.
- When reconstituting a powder injectable, the powder must be soluble in the diluent. Sterile water is a commonly used diluent. Remember to always check the insert to make sure the drug is soluble in the diluents before mixing.

Adsorption

Adsorption occurs when a CSP in gas or liquid form accumulates on the surface of a solid or liquid. For example, insulin adsorption on the surfaces of IV containers is a problem. As insulin is adsorbed, its concentration in the solution goes down. Adsorption issues can be addressed by adjusting the amount of drug injected into the solution such that the correct amount of drug is in available in the solution to be delivered via the IV tubing.

Absorption

Absorption occurs when a material or container soaks up all or part of a liquid CSP. For example, glass is used to store nitroglycerin because soft plastic containers absorb the liquid and glass does not. Likewise, when you make an IV using nitroglycerin you put it in a glass IV bottle so that you don't lose any of the drug, which would be absorbed into a plastic IV bag.

Color Change

Color change occurs when the original color of one or more products in a mixture changes. For example, a combination of dobutamine and nitroglycerin will change to a pale pink solution. If you add sodium nitroprusside to the solution and expose it to light, you will get a pale pink solution with a small amount of dark brown precipitate.

Separation

Sometimes when preparing a product, the ingredients will separate out in the mixture. This is sometimes found in a 3:1 TPN. A 3:1 TPN contains amino acids, dextrose and lipids in one bag. Because this is a mixture of oil and water, they will sometimes separate in the IV bag. Depending on the situation, the result may be:

- Creaming—accumulation of triglyceride molecules at the top of the emulsion
- Aggregation—clumping of triglycerides molecules within the emulsion
- Coalescence—fusion of small triglyceride particles into larger ones

- Cracking—separation of the oil and water components of the emulsion

(TPNs will be further discussed in Chapter 8.)

Chemical Incompatibility

Sometimes, when two products are combined, a chemical change occurs. This changes the properties of the products. As a result, the action and effectiveness of the products changes, too. Pharmacy technicians must know which CSPs are chemically incompatible.

When products are chemically incompatible, one of the following reactions may take place:

- Hydrolysis—when hydrolysis occurs, a product combines with water, and two new products form. Hydrolysis changes the properties of the original product(s).
- Oxidation/reduction—when products go through an oxidation/reduction reaction, one product loses electrons and the other gains electrons. This seemingly tiny change alters the chemical properties of the products.
- Photolysis—photolysis happens when a product breaks down after exposure to light. Once photolysis occurs, the original product is irreversibly changed. One example of this is nitroprusside. When sodium nitroprusside is put into an IV bag, it must be protected from light. If not, the solution will turn orange, dark brown or blue. A blue solution is almost totally degraded.

T I P You should always check package inserts for information about possible incompatibilities. Additional sources of information include *Handbook of Injectable Drugs* (Trissel), *Stability of Compounded Formulations* (Trissel), *King's Guide to Parenteral Admixtures*, *Extended Stability for Parenteral Drugs* (Bing), American Journal of Health-System Pharmacy, and other primary literature journals.

pH, Acids, and Bases

One reason for keeping products free of contamination is to maintain the pH level. When a product becomes contaminated, its pH may be changed. This in turn changes the properties of that product. The pH is also important because it affects how products react when they are combined.

The **pH** of a substance describes how acidic or basic it is. The pH scale ranges from 0 (very acidic) to 14 (very basic, or alkaline). The middle of the pH scale is 7.0, which is neutral. Human blood has a pH of 7.4, just above neutral, or slightly basic. The outside surface of the eye has a pH of 6.5 to 7.6. Parts of the digestive system can have a pH as high as 8.0 or as low as 0.7! Figure 2-2 shows the pH of several familiar substances.

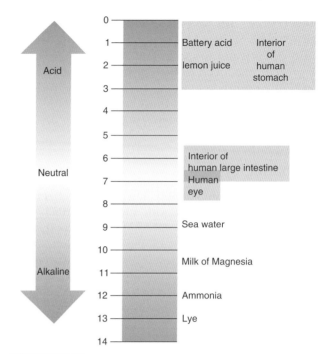

FIGURE 2-2 pH scale.

The pH of CSPs becomes critically important when:

- CSPs are combined or mixed together, or a CSP is combined with another product. If the pH of all products being combined is not compatible, the pH of one or all products will change.
- CSPs come into contact with the body. The pH of the body tissue and the pH of the CSP must be compatible. If they are not, pain may result.

Always remember, if the pH of a CSP changes, its properties may change.

Buffers

A **buffer** is a compound or mixture of compounds that helps prevent changes in pH. As you now know, if the pH of a product changes, its properties may change. Buffers help keep this from happening. Here are some examples:

- A buffer is added to a CSP. The presence of the buffer helps prevent tissue damage or pain that would otherwise result when certain CSPs are applied to sensitive membranes or nasal passages; it is injected into muscles, organs, or injury sites.
- A buffer is added to a solution in which certain CSPs are dissolved. The buffer maintains the solution's pH and the chemical stability of the solution.

Types of Buffers

Typical buffers include:

- boric acid solution (ophthalmic solutions, or solutions used in the eye)
- sodium bicarbonate

- weak hydrochloric acid
- weak sodium hydroxide solution

Routes of Administration

The type of buffer used depends on the drug's route of administration—the path a drug follows as it comes into contact with the body. For instance, certain buffers can only be used for ophthalmic solutions (solutions administered in the eye) because they are toxic if used systemically. A buffer is used to keep the pH of a solution or product compatible with its route of administration. Here are some examples of typical routes of administration:

- applied directly to a lesion or wound
- injected into the circulatory system, muscle tissue, or heart
- applied or injected into the eye or ear
- taken by mouth
- inhaled into the nasal passages
- administered through a feeding tube into the digestive system

Because the pH of human blood is around 7.4, a CSP injected into the circulatory system must be compatible. Buffers can help achieve a compatible pH. On the other hand, the pH inside the eyeball is 7.5 to 7.6. The outside surface of the eyeball can be as low as 6.5. As you can see, ophthalmic CSPs must be buffered to match the sites where they are administered.

TIP Unlike water, contact lens solution is isotonic—it has the same osmolarity as the tissue and cells of the outside eye area.

Tonicity

Another property that applies to CSPs in solution is tonicity. **Tonicity** describes the way cells and tissues react to a solution that surrounds them. The term is specific to situations in which a semi-permeable membrane separates one solution from another.

For example, an open wound is often cleaned and bathed with saline solution. A membrane surrounds each cell in the wound area. When saline solution is applied, the cells become bathed or immersed in the solution. Depending on the tonicity of the solution, water moves across the membrane in one direction or another.

Three types of tonicity describe the direction in which water and solutes move: hypertonic, hypotonic, and isotonic.

Hypertonic

A hypertonic solution contains more solutes per solvent than the cells it surrounds. When cells are surrounded by a hypertonic solution, osmotic pressure forces water to move out of the cells and into the solution. This action causes the cells to shrivel.

Hypotonic

A hypotonic solution contains fewer solutes per solvent than the cells it surrounds. When cells are surrounded by a hypotonic solution, osmotic pressure forces water to move from the solution into the cell. This causes the cells to swell or even burst.

Isotonic

An isotonic solution contains the same amount of solutes per solvent as the cells it surrounds. When cells are surrounded by an isotonic solution, there is no osmotic pressure. Therefore, the movement of water and solutes is stable and cells neither shrink nor swell.

The body's isotonic solutions fall between 280 and 310 milliosmoles per liter. Knowing the tonicity of the body area into which an IV CSP solution is to be administered is critical. CSP solutions given by IV should be isotonic.

Osmolality and Osmolarity

Two other properties of CSPs are **osmolality** and **osmolarity**.

- Osmolality is the number of osmoles of solute per kilogram of solvent (mOsm/kg).
- Osmolarity is the number of osmoles of solute per liter of solution (mOsm/L).

Remember that tonicity is the *relative* measure of the movement of water between two solutions. Osmolarity, on the other hand, is not a *relative* measure, but an *absolute* measure of osmotically active solutes in a solution.

When you know and understand the osmolarity of a solution, you avoid potential problems with the administration of IV solutions. There are many ways to calculate the osmolarity of a solution. The details for making these calculations will be discussed in Chapter 3.

CHAPTER HIGHLIGHTS

- Contamination of CSPs can happen through physical contamination (including touch contamination, and shadowing), or microbial contamination.
- Touch contamination occurs when physical contact occurs between an object and a CSP.
- Shadowing happens when the HEPA filtered airflow in a hooded work area is blocked to a critical site.
- Microbial contamination can be minimized when preparing CSPs by proper hand scrubbing, wearing protective garb and gloves, covering facial and head hair, and abstaining from talking, eating, chewing gum and drinking.
- Stability describes the ability of a CSP to stay effective until it is used or until its expiration or beyond-use date.
- CSPs are commonly stored in designated refrigerators, freezers, or locked cabinets.

- The beyond-use date is the date after which a CSP should not be used. It is determined by the pharmacist and found on the pharmacy prepared label affixed to the IV the container.
- The pharmacist determines the beyond-use date, and the manufacturer determines the expiration date.
- Compatibility and incompatibility describes how well or poorly one product combines with another product.
- Types of physical incompatibility include precipitate, giving off heat or cold, changing color, and becoming cloudy. Types of chemical incompatibility include hydrolysis, photolysis, oxidation/reduction, adsorption, and absorption.
- If the pH of a CSP changes, its physical and chemical properties may change. This may affect the stability of the CSP, as well as its compatibility with other products.
- Hypertonic describes a solution that contains more solutes per solvent than the cells it surrounds. Hypotonic describes a solution that contains fewer solutes per solvent than the cells it surrounds. Isotonic describes a solution that contains the same amount of solutes per solvent as the cells it surrounds.
- A hypertonic CSP solution given intravenously causes the cells of the body to shrink. A hypotonic CSP solution causes the body cells to swell.
- Osmotic pressure is the pressure produced by either a hypertonic or hypotonic solution.
- Osmolarity and osmolality describe the solute concentrate of a solution.

QUICK QUIZ

Answer the following multiple-choice questions.

1. What occurs if fibers from your clothing fall into a CSP?
   a. microbial contamination
   b. shadowing
   c. touch contamination
   d. chemical incompatibility
2. In which location would shadowing most likely occur?
   a. in a CSP storage cabinet
   b. in an LAFW
   c. in a designated CSP freezer
   d. in a nonsterile preparation area
3. The beyond-use date is determined by the
   a. pharmacist.
   b. medical doctor.
   c. manufacturer.
   d. patient.
4. Which of the following indicates physical incompatibility in a CSP?
   a. photolysis
   b. oxidation/reduction
   c. hydrolysis
   d. precipitation
5. Body cells immersed in a hypotonic solution will:
   a. remain stable.
   b. shrink.
   c. swell.
   d. precipitate.

Please answer each of the following questions in one to three sentences.

1. Explain the difference between a critical site and a critical area.

   _____

   _____

2. What are contaminants and how do they affect CSPs?

   _____

   _____

3. How can pharmacy technicians help prevent microbial contamination of CSPs?

   _____

   _____

4. A CSP is administered into the circulatory system. What pH should the CSP have? Why?

   _____

   _____

5. What does the osmolarity of a solution tell you? Why is this important?

   _____

   _____

Answer the following questions as either true or false.

1. ____ The higher the osmolarity of a solution, the more concentrated it is.
2. ____ An area of turbulence occurs when the airflow in an LAFW becomes blocked.
3. ____ Particles and fibers from clothing are examples of microbial contamination.
4. ____ A pH of 12.5 indicates a substance is an acid.
5. ____ Precipitation is a sign of physical incompatibility.

Match the term in the left column with the correct description from the right column.

1. expiration date	a. triangular-shaped area behind an object placed in a LAFW
2. area of turbulence	b. determined by manufacturer
3. adsorption	c. used to make pH compatible
4. absorption	d. a CSP accumulates on a surface
5. buffer	e. a CSP is soaked up by the IV container

CHAPTER 3

Sterile Product Calculations

- Calculate the concentration of a CSP based on a medication order.
- Calculate the correct dose of a CSP based on body weight and body surface area.
- Calculate the amount of concentrated sodium chloride needed to make a fractional saline CSP.
- Calculate the amount of diluent and powder volume for a CSP that is to be reconstituted.
- Calculate dilutions using the alligation method.
- Calculate the osmolarity of a CSP.
- Calculate the flow rate of a CSP based on a medication order.

KEY TERMS

ABW—actual body weight
active ingredient—the substance or chemical responsible for the action of the finished product
alligation—the calculation of the relative amount of ingredients of different percentage strengths to make up a product of a given strength
BSA—body surface area
D5W—dextrose 5% in water; commonly used base solution for CSPs
daily dose—the amount of a drug to be taken over 24 hours
diluent—a product that is added to a solution to reduce its strength, or dilute it
dimensional analysis—a problem-solving method in which any number or expression can be multiplied by one without changing its value
IBW—ideal body weight
infusion pump—an automatic device used with an IV system for delivering medication at regular intervals in specific quantities

IPA—isopropyl alcohol
isotonic solution—a solution with an osmotic pressure equal to that of the inside of a body cell
LBW—lean body weight
loading dose—a large initial dose required to achieve the desired blood drug level given at the beginning of a therapeutic regimen
maintenance dose—a smaller dose following the loading dose to sustain the desired drug blood level or drug effect
narrow therapeutic index (NTI)—small room for error
nomogram—a chart that uses the patient's height and weight to estimate the body surface area in square meters
normal saline (NS)—an isotonic solution containing 0.9% sodium chloride; commonly used base solution for CSPs
powder volume—the volume that a powder occupies after it is dissolved in a solution
reconstitution—the process in which a diluent is added to a powered form of a drug
w/v—weight/volume

As a pharmacy technician, you will receive orders for various concentrations, amounts, and mixtures of CSPs. In many cases, the exact concentrations or mixtures ordered will not be available. When this happens, you'll need to know how to combine precise quantities and accurate concentration strengths to make the final CSP. This assures that the patient gets the right drug in the right amount.

In this chapter, you'll learn how to calculate the concentration of one or more ingredients used to prepare a CSP. You'll also learn how to obtain a solution with a specific concentration and how to reconstitute powders to a given dilution. In addition, you'll understand how to calculate osmolarity of an IV admixture, as well as how to calculate flow rates.

UNDERSTANDING CONCENTRATIONS

Concentration provides the quantity of the **active ingredient** per amount of product or preparation. An active ingredient is a chemical or substance that is responsible for the action of the finished product. The amount may be expressed as volume or weight.

Concentrations are always used for expressing doses for topical preparations. In this case, the concentration is the driving force for transfer of the drug across the skin. Concentration is also used to express the strength of liquid systemic products, such as IV admixtures. For example:

- amoxicillin 250 mg/5 mL
- dextrose 5% in water

LITER CONCENTRATION CALCULATIONS

When you prepare an IV admixture, the guideline to follow is usually the concentration of a particular active ingredient per a particular volume of solution. Many IV admixtures contain one or more active ingredients. Since reference materials and the literature often use a standard concentration, it is important that you are able to easily convert concentrations. Often, the concentration is expressed in grams/liter. However, at other times the concentration is expressed in mg/mL. If you cannot easily convert between grams and milligrams or liters and milliliters, then you should review those calculations. Remember that there are 1000 milligrams in 1 gram and 1000 milliliters in 1 liter.

The solutions in which the ingredients are dissolved are typically normal saline (NS) or dextrose 5% in water (**D5W**). **Normal saline** is an isotonic solution containing 0.9% sodium chloride.

In most cases, you'll have to determine the concentration of a CSP based on a medication order. The following examples show how to determine the amount of active ingredient that has been added to a liter of IV solution.

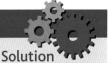

SAMPLE CALCULATIONS

Active Ingredient Added to IV Solution

Example 1
Calculate the concentration of ampicillin in the following order in grams/liter: Ampicillin 400 mg in 50 mL NS

Step 1. *Start with what you know.*
Ampicillin 400 mg in 50 mL NS

Step 2. *Convert mL to L.*

$$\frac{400mg}{50mL} \times \frac{1{,}000mL}{L} = \frac{400{,}000mg}{50L} = \frac{Xmg}{L}$$

Step 3. *Cross-multiply.*

$$\frac{400{,}000mg}{50L} = \frac{Xmg}{L}$$

$$50X = 400{,}000 \times 1$$
$$50X = 400{,}000$$

Step 4. *Divide to find X.*
Divide both sides by 50:

$$X = \frac{400{,}000}{50}$$

$$X = 8{,}000$$
$$X = 8{,}000 \text{ mg/L or } 8 \text{ mg/mL}$$

Therefore, the concentration of the final product is 8000 mg of ampicillin per liter, or 8 milligrams of ampicillin per milliliter of normal saline.

Example 2
Calculate the concentration of cefazolin in the following order in mg/mL: Cefazolin 750 mg in 100 mL D5W

Step 1. *Start with what you know.*
Cefazolin 750 mg in 100 mL D5W

Step 2. *Convert mL to L.*

$$\frac{750mg}{100mL} \times \frac{1000mL}{L} = \frac{750{,}000mg}{100L} = \frac{Xmg}{L}$$

Step 3. *Cross-multiply.*

$$\frac{750{,}000mg}{100L} = \frac{Xmg}{L}$$

$$100X = 750{,}000 \times 1$$
$$100X = 750{,}000$$

Step 4. *Divide to find X.*
Divide both sides by 100:

$$X = \frac{750{,}000}{100}$$

$$X = 7500$$
$$X = 7500 \text{ mg/L or } 7.5 \text{ mg/mL}$$

Therefore, the concentration of the final product is 7500 mg of cefazolin per liter of D5W, or 7.5 mg of cefazolin per milliliter of D5W.

Example 3
Calculate the concentration of heparin in the following order: Heparin 10,000 units in 250 mL D5W

Step 1. *Start with what you know.*
Heparin 10,000 units in 250 mL D5W

Step 2. *Convert mL to L.*

$$\frac{10{,}000U}{250mL} \times \frac{100mL}{L} = \frac{10{,}000{,}000U}{250L} = \frac{XU}{L}$$

Step 3. *Cross-multiply.*

$$\frac{10,000,000U}{250L} = \frac{XU}{L}$$

$$250X = 10,000,000 \times 1$$
$$250X = 10,000,000$$

Step 4. *Divide to find X.*
Divide both sides by 250:

$$X = \frac{10,000,000}{250}$$
$$X = 40,000$$
$$X = 40,000 \text{ U/L or } 40 \text{ U/mL}$$

Therefore, the concentration of the final product is 40 units of heparin per milliliter of D5W, or 40,000 units of heparin per liter of D5W.

TIP After the concentration is confirmed, you can use Trissel's *Handbook of Injectable Drugs* and the package insert to determine any stability issues. Remember from Chapter 2 that the loss of stability affects the properties and effectiveness of a product.

DOSAGE CALCULATIONS

Once you've calculated the concentration of your product, your next step is to evaluate the order for dosing accuracy. One of your most critical tasks as a pharmacy technician is to make sure patients get the right drug in the right amount.

There are various accepted methods of determining dosage amounts. These are based on:

- actual body weight
- ideal body weight
- body surface area
- simple equations

Regardless of the method, you should always double-check the dose and dosage regimen to verify accuracy and appropriateness.

Dosage Expression

Before you can calculate the dosage of a medication, you must know how dosages are expressed. Individual doses are expressed using one of the following formats:

- quantity of drug (for example, 25 mg)
- quantity of drug per kilogram of patient body weight (for example, 5 mg drug/kg body weight)
- quantity of drug per square meter of patient body surface area **(BSA)** (for example, 10 mg drug/m² of the BSA)

 PROCEED WITH CAUTION

Toxic Dosing

Even small changes in NTI drugs, such as chemotherapy agents, could have toxic results. Dosing based on body weight provides accurate indications for dosing. This only works, however, if you obtain the *accurate* body weight.

Dosage Based on Body Weight

The calculation methods for doses that are based on the patient's body weight are based on *actual* body weight or *ideal* body weight. Methods based on body weight are often used for pediatric doses. A typical pediatric medication order would specify the child's weight, for example, 70 lb.

Methods based on body weight are also important when determining adult doses for drugs that have a **narrow therapeutic index (NTI)**, or small room for error.

Actual Body Weight of Adults

When a prescription or medication drug order is written in terms of a quantity (micrograms, milligrams, grams, etc.) per kilogram or pound of body weight, you must determine the **ABW**, or actual body weight, from one of the following sources:

- the prescriber/physician
- the patient
- the patient's caregiver

You use the ABW to check the prescribed dose for appropriateness and in calculating the intended dose.

Actual Body Weight of Pediatric Patients

You can perform initial dosing checks for pediatric patients without the ABW if the child's age is known. In this case you'd base the dose on an estimate of body weight. You can use a percentile chart of body weight versus age to find this estimate.

Ideal Body Weight

For some types of patients, such as those who are obese, dosing is based on estimated **IBW**, or ideal body weight. Ideal body weight is often referred to as **LBW**, or lean body weight. The pharmacist will be able to direct you when an IBW should be used in the dosage calculation. The following equations are used to calculate estimated IBW in kilograms:

- *adult males:*

$$IBW_{(kg)} = 50 + (2.3 \times \text{height in inches over five feet})$$

- *adult females:*

$$IBW_{(kg)} = 45.5 + (2.3 \times \text{height in inches over five feet})$$

- *children under five feet tall:*

$$IBW_{(kg)} = \frac{height^2_{cm} \times 1.65}{1000}$$

- *children 5 feet and taller:*

males: $IBW_{(kg)} = 39 + (2.27 \times height_{(in)}$ over 5 feet)
females: $IBW_{(kg)} = 42.2 + (2.27 \times height_{(in)}$ over 5 feet)

Dosing Based on Body Surface Area

A drug dose may also be based on estimated BSA. A dosage based on BSA is expressed as a quantity of the drug per square meter of BSA.

You might use a patient's BSA when the dosage depends on a patient's height and weight, or length for an infant. Dosing based on BSA is the most accurate method for children up to 12 years of age and for adults who are below normal body weight.

You can use either nomograms or simple equations to find a patient's BSA.

Nomograms to Find BSA

One method to obtain the BSA is by using a **nomogram**. A nomogram is a chart that uses the patient's height and weight to estimate the body surface area in square meters (see nomograms in Appendix C). A straight line is drawn from the patient's height in inches or centimeters (in the left column) to the patient's weight in kilograms or pounds (in the right column). The point where the line intersects the middle column is the patient's BSA.

T I P If a nomogram reads 68 cm for height and 72 kg for weight, the BSA is 1.36 m². Nomograms are incredibly useful tools.

After you determine the patient's estimated BSA, use the following formula to calculate a child's dose:

(BSA × adult dose) ÷ 1.7 = child's dose

Using Equations to Find BSA

The BSA can also be calculated using two basic equations.

- Using weight in pounds and height in inches:

$$BSA(m^2) = \sqrt{\frac{Ht(in) \times Wt(lb)}{3131}}$$

- Using weight in kilograms and height in centimeters:

$$BSA(m^2) = \sqrt{\frac{Ht(cm) \times Wt(kg)}{3600}}$$

Calculations of Quantities

In addition to determining dosages based on patient's weight or surface area, you'll be required to determine various size doses based on different medication orders and dosing regimens. In most cases, you'll have to calculate these doses based on what you have in stock.

Calculating Loading Dose

A **loading dose** is a large initial dose required to achieve the desired blood drug level given at the start of a therapeutic regimen. Pharmacy technicians who work in a hospital setting often calculate loading doses.

For example, a patient with heart failure may be prescribed digoxin. The medication order might be as follows:

"Heart failure: (intravenous and/or oral capsule) for rapid digitalization, give loading dose of 0.4 to 0.6 mg IV; additional doses of 0.1 to 0.3 mg IV may be given cautiously at 6 to 8 hr intervals if necessary to achieve response."

Here is an example of calculating a loading dose:

Medication order: Ciprofloxacin hydrochloride 1 g po now
Available: Duricef (cefadroxil) 500 mg/5 mL

Step 1. *Convert grams to milligrams by cross-multiplying.*

$$\frac{1g}{1000mg} = \frac{1g}{Xmg}$$

1X = 1000 × 1
1X = 1000

Step 2. *Divide to find X.*
Divide both sides by 1:

$$\frac{X = 1000}{1}$$

X = 1000

Step 3. *Cross-multiply.*

$$\frac{100mg}{5mL} = \frac{1000mg}{X}$$

100X = 1000 × 5
100X = 5000

Step 4. *Divide to find X.*
Divide both sides by 100:

$$\frac{X = 5000}{100}$$

X = 50

Therefore, the loading dose of 1 g cefadroxil = 50 mL.

Calculating the Daily Dose

The **daily dose** is the amount of a drug to be taken over 24 hours. Most of the time, the daily dose is considered the **maintenance dose**—a smaller dose following the loading dose administered to sustain the desired drug blood level or drug effect.

Following is an example of how to calculate a typical daily dose as a maintenance dose to follow the loading dose provided in the previous section.

Medication order: 0.5 g q12h × 10 days
Available: Duricef® (cefadroxil) 500 mg/5 mL

Step 1. *Convert grams to milligrams by cross multiplying.*

$$\frac{1}{500} = \frac{1}{X}$$

$$1X = 1 \times 500$$
$$1X = 500$$

Step 2. *Divide.*
Divide both sides by 1 to find X:

$$X = \frac{500}{1}$$

$$X = 500$$
So, 0.5 g = 500 mg.

Step 3. *Calculate the daily dose.*

The available form is 500 mg per 5 mL. Therefore, each dose after the loading dose will be 5 mL.

Let's take a look at a couple more calculations. In these, you'll see how an actual medication order may appear from a physician.

SAMPLE CALCULATIONS

Dosing

Example 1
Calculate the number of 100 mg capsules required for the following order: Dilantin 300 mg daily for 1 month.

Step 1. *No conversion necessary.*

Step 2. *Set up the problem.*

$$\frac{100mg}{1cap} = \frac{300mg}{X}$$

Step 3. *Cross-multiply.*

$$\frac{100}{1} = \frac{300}{X}$$

$$100X = 300 \times 1$$
$$100X = 300$$

Step 4. *Divide.*
Divide both sides by 100:

$$X = \frac{300}{100}$$

$$X = 3$$

Assuming there are 30 days in a month, 30 (days) × 3 (capsules) = 90. Therefore, you must dispense 90 capsules to the patient.

Example 2
A physician prescribed a patient Septra DS—a combination drug containing 160 mg of trimethoprim and 800 mg of sulfamethoxazole. However, this patient has a hard time swallowing tablets and prefers to take a liquid form if one is available. Trimethoprim/sulfamethoxazole suspension contains 40 mg trimethoprim and 200 mg sulfamethoxazole in 5 mL. Calculate (in milliliters) the amount that must be dispensed for the patient to complete this regimen: Septra DSiq12h × 10 days.

Step 1. *Set up problem for the first ingredient.*
160 mg of liquid trimethoprim is needed. The liquid formulation contains 40 mg of trimethoprim/5 mL:

$$\frac{40mg}{5mL} = \frac{160mg}{XmL}$$

Step 2. *Calculate the first problem by cross-multiplying.*

$$\frac{40mg}{5mL} = \frac{160mg}{XmL}$$

$$40X = 160 \times 5$$
$$40X = 800$$

Step 3. *Divide.*
Divide both sides by 40:

$$X = \frac{800}{40}$$

$$X = 20$$

Step 4. *Set up the problem for the second ingredient.*
800 mg of liquid sulfamethoxazole is needed. The liquid formulation contains 200 mg/5 mL.

$$\frac{200mg}{5mL} = \frac{800mg}{X}$$

Step 5. *Calculate the second problem by cross-multiplying.*

$$\frac{200}{5} = \frac{800}{X}$$

$$200X = 800 \times 5$$
$$200X = 4000$$

Step 6. *Divide.*
Divide both sides by 200.

$$X = \frac{4000}{200}$$

$$X = 20 \text{ mL}$$

Therefore, 20 mL of the liquid preparation is needed to equal one tablet of the Septra DS.

Step 7. *Label the product in a household measure.*
5 mL = 1 tsp, therefore, 20 mL = 4 tsp per dose. Every 12 hours indicates two doses per day: 20 mL × 2 = 40 mL daily × 10 days = 400 mL of Septra suspension to give 10 days' worth.

Therefore, you must dispense 400 mL of Septra to the patient.

FRACTIONAL SALINE CALCULATIONS

At times, a physician will order that a medication be placed in a base solution that you do not normally stock. A common example of this is a fractional saline, such as D5 ¼ NS or D5 ½ NS. If the pharmacy does not stock these solutions, then you will need to make them from what is already in stock.

You could use a bag of D5W and a bag of NS to make a fractional saline. However, if you do the math you will quickly learn that it will take large volumes of each solution to get the desired concentration. You need to check the pharmacy stock and see what concentration sodium chloride you have in stock. Two common concentrations are 23.4% and 14.6% sodium chloride. Following are some examples.

SAMPLE CALCULATIONS

Fractional Solutions

Example 1
The pharmacy only stocks D5W. How much concentrated (e.g., 14.6%) NaCl would be used to make D5 ½NS?

Step 1. *Start with what you have.*
14.6% NaCl

Step 2. *Figure out what you need.*
1L (1000 mL) of D5W ½NS (0.45% NaCl)

Step 3. *Restate the problem.*
How much 14.6% NaCl do I add to a liter bag of D5W to make D5W ½ NS?

Step 4. *Put the information you know into the problem.*
X mL × 14.6% NaCl = 1000 mL × 0.45% NaCl

Step 5. *Cross-multiply.*
$$\frac{X\,mL}{1000\,mL} = \frac{0.0045}{0.146}$$
$$X = 1000\ mL \times 0.0045$$

Step 6. *Divide.*
Divide both sides by 0.146.
$$\frac{X = 4.5}{0.146}$$
$$X = 30.82\ mL$$

Therefore, add 30.82 mL of 14.6% NaCl to a liter bag of D5W make D5W ½NS.

Example 2
The pharmacy only stocks D5W. How much concentrated 23.4% NaCl would be used to make D5 ½NS?

Step 1. *Start with what you have.*
23.4% NaCl

Step 2. *Figure out what you need.*
1 L (1000 mL) of D5W ½NS

Step 3. *Restate the problem.*
How much 23.4% NaCl do you add to a liter bag of D5W to make D5W ½NS?

Step 4. *Put the information you know into the problem.*
X mL × 23.4% NaCl = 1000 mL × 0.45% NaCl

Step 5. *Cross-multiply.*
$$\frac{0.0234}{1000\,mL} = \frac{0.0045}{X}$$
$$0.234X = 1000 \times 0.0045$$
$$0.234X = 4.5$$

Step 6. *Divide.*
Divide both sides by 0.234.
$$\frac{X = 4.5}{0.234}$$
$$X = 19.23\ mL$$

Therefore, add 19.23 mL of 23.4% NaCl to a liter bag of D5W to make D5W ½NS.

RECONSTITUTING POWDERS

Some parenteral drugs have limited stability when in solution. For this reason, some products are lyophilized, or freeze-dried, and come from the manufacturer in powder form for reconstitution.

Reconstitution is the process in which a diluent is added to the powder. A **diluent**, or solvent, is something that is added to a product to reduce its strength, or dilute it. Sterile water and sterile sodium chloride are common examples of diluents.

Understanding Powder Volume

The volume that the powder occupies after it is dissolved in a solution is called the **powder volume**. The volume of most lyophilized powders is so small that in most cases, you can disregard it when making calculations.

In other products, the powder may occupy a much larger volume. In this case, you must account for the powder volume when making calculations involving concentrated solutions.

The final volume of the reconstituted product is the volume of the diluent plus the volume of the powder.

Instructions for reconstitution are often included on the package label. If they are not there, then they can be found in the package insert from the manufacturer. One important thing to keep in mind when reconstituting powders: if a powder takes up volume, then it must be taken into account when doing calculations. Often the package insert will disregard powder volume if it is assumed that the entire volume in the vial will be used. Read all of the reconstitution instructions carefully and take powder volume into consideration when preparing all reconstitutions.

Reconstitution to a Set Dilution

To ensure accuracy, many organizations set standards of dosing because each drug has a different powder volume. These standards might call for specific concentrations regardless of the manufacturer's instructions for reconstitution.

Here's an example of how to calculate a reconstitution based on a set dilution.

Let's say a hospital has a policy that all reconstitutions have a resulting concentration of 100 mg/mL. You must reconstitute a 1 gram vial of nafcillin. According to the package information if you add 3.4 mL of diluent, you'll end up with a concentration of 250 mg/mL. But you must follow hospital policy so that the resulting concentration is 100 mg/mL.

With these restrictions in mind, how do you dilute the 250 mg/mL to 100 mg/mL?

Step 1. *Restate the problem.*

If you add 3.4 mL of diluent to a 1 gram vial of nafcillin, you will have a resulting concentration of 250 mg/mL.

Step 2. Determine the resulting volume if reconstituted per package instructions.

If the concentration is 250 mg/mL and you have 1 gram (1000 milligrams) in the vial, then you should have 4 mL of solution after dilution.

$$\frac{250\,mg}{1\,mL} = \frac{1000\,mg}{X\,mL}$$

X = 4 mL

Step 3. Determine powder volume

If you have 4 mL in the vial after reconstitution and you put 3.4 mL of diluent in the vial, then 4 − 3.4 = 0.6 mL is the volume taken up by the powder.

Step 4. Determine the resulting volume at a concentration of 100 mg/mL.

$$\frac{100\,mg}{1\,mL} = \frac{1000\,mg}{X\,mL}$$

X = 10 mL

Step 5. Determine the amount of diluent that will be needed.

Final volume at concentration of 100 mg/mL − powder volume = amount of diluent needed

10 mL − 0.6 mL = 9.4 mL diluent needed

Therefore, you dilute this suspension to a concentration of 100 mg/mL by adding 9.4 mL of diluent.

ALLIGATION

A common task of a pharmacy technician is to use two products of different percentage strengths to prepare a third product with a desired concentration. An easy way to do this is by using the alligation method.

Alligation is the calculation of the relative amount of ingredients of different percentage strengths to make up a product of a given strength. You may use diluents when making these products. Remember that diluents are substances with no active ingredient, and therefore, are at 0% concentration. Active ingredients alone are 100% concentration. Remember you must have one product more concentrated and one product less concentrated than your desired product.

Let's work through a couple examples of calculations using the alligation method.

SAMPLE CALCULATIONS

Alligation

Example 1
You need to make 120 mL of a 50% solution of **IPA** (isopropyl alcohol). But the only ingredients you have on hand are 100% IPA and water. You need to know how many milliliters of each ingredient to use to make the 50% IPA.

Step 1. *Start with what you have.*
100% IPA and water (0%)

Step 2. *Figure out what you need.*
120 mL of 50% IPA

Step 3. *Use an alligation diagram to determine how much of each ingredient to use.*

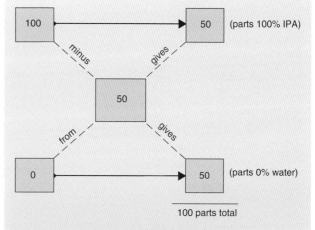

Based on the alligation figure above, you should be able to determine what you need to make this solution:

- 50% IPA in equal parts—50 parts of each for a proportion of 1:1
- 60 mL of IPA and 60 mL of water

Sample calculations continues on pg. 24

Example 2

This time, you need to prepare 4500 mL of a 10% **w/v**, or weight/volume, dextrose solution. You have 50% w/v dextrose and 5% w/v dextrose.

Step 1. *Start with what you have.*
50% w/v dextrose solution and 5% w/v dextrose solution

Step 2. *Figure out what you need.*
4500 mL 10% w/v dextrose

Step 3. *Use an alligation diagram to determine how much of each ingredient to use.*

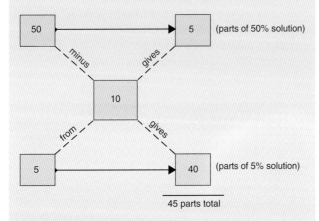

(parts of 50% solution)

(parts of 5% solution)

45 parts total

In this situation, you have a proportion of 40:5, or 8:1, for a total of 9 parts. Therefore, you need to mix eight parts of 5% dextrose with one part of 50% dextrose. To find the total amount of 5% dextrose and 50% dextrose you need for a 4500-mL solution, follow these steps:

Step 4. *Set up a proportion for the first ingredient (50% dextrose).*

$$\frac{9\,parts}{1\,part} = \frac{4500\,mL}{X\,mL}$$

Step 5. *Cross-multiply.*

$$\frac{9}{1} = \frac{4500}{X}$$

$$9X = 4500 \times 1$$
$$9X = 4500$$

Step 6. *Divide.*
Divide both sides by 9.

$$X = \frac{4500}{9}$$

X = 500 of 50% dextrose solution

Step 7. *Set up the problem for the second ingredient (5% dextrose).*

$$\frac{9\,parts}{8\,parts} = \frac{4500\,mL}{Y\,mL}$$

Step 8. *Cross-multiply.*

$$\frac{9}{8} = \frac{4500}{Y}$$

$$9Y = 4500 \times 8$$
$$9Y = 36{,}000$$

Step 9. *Divide.*
Divide both sides by 9.

$$Y = \frac{36{,}000}{9}$$

Y = 4000 of 5% dextrose solution

Therefore, you need 500 mL of 50% dextrose solution and 4000 mL of 5% dextrose solution.

TONICITY CALCULATIONS

To make sure an injected CSP does not cause an adverse reaction, the tonicity, osmolality, and osmolarity of the solution must always be considered.

You learned a bit about these terms in Chapter 2. Let's review before you learn how to calculate osmolarity.

Tonicity

The tonicity of a solution is the measure of particles in a solution compared to that of a certain cell type. Solutions can be isotonic, hypertonic, or hypotonic.

- An **isotonic solution** has an osmotic pressure equal to that of the inside of the cell.
- A **hypotonic** solution has an osmotic pressure lower than that of the inside of the cell.
- A **hypertonic** solution has an osmotic pressure greater than that of the inside of the cell.

Osmolarity

Remember that osmolarity is the exact measure of particles in a solution per unit of solution, expressed as milliosmoles per liter, or mOsm/L. Osmolality is simply the number of particles of a solution per kilogram of solution, expressed as mOsm/kg).

The normal osmolarity of blood is between 300 and 310 mOsm/L. You should try to match the osmolarity as closely as possible when you prepare pharmaceutical solutions that are administered parenterally or applied topically to sensitive membranes, such as the eye.

T I P For most adults, the lining of the gastrointestinal tract can tolerate highly hypertonic solutions (those of high osmolarity). In contrast, the gastrointestinal lining of infants is sensitive to hypertonic solutions. Oral solutions for infants should have a lower osmolarity—close to 300 mOsmol/L.

Calculating Osmolarity

Calculating the osmolarity of a CSP admixture is easy, but first you must know the osmolarity and volume of each individual ingredient. Usually, this information can be found on the package insert.

Once you know the osmolarity and volume of each ingredient, you are ready to calculate the total osmolarity of solution. There are many ways to do this. The example below uses a simple four- step method for a typical IV admixture.

Find the total osmolarity of an admixture containing the following ingredients:

- sterile water
- sodium bicarbonate
- potassium acetate
- folic acid
- pyridoxine
- calcium chloride

Step 1. *Multiply.*

Multiply the volume in milliliters of each ingredient times its osmolarity.

Sterile water—500 mL × 0.00 = 0.00
Sodium bicarbonate—50 mL × 2.00 = 100.00
Potassium acetate—10 mL × 4.00 = 40.00
Folic acid—0.5 mL × 0.20 = 0.10
Pyridoxine—1 mL × 1.11 = 1.11
Calcium chloride—1 mL × 2.04 = 2.04

Step 2. *Add.*

Add the *products* from Step 1. This gives the total mOsmol/L in the solution.

```
   0.00
 100.00
  40.00
   0.20
   1.11
+  2.04
-------
 143.25
```

Total mOsm/L = 143.2

Step 3. *Add again!*

Add together the *volume* of each ingredient in the solution. This gives the total volume of the mixture.

```
 500 mL
  50 mL
  10 mL
 0.5 mL
   1 mL
+  1 mL
-------
562.5 mL
```

Total volume = 562.5 mL

Step 4. *Divide.*

Finally, divide the total milliosmoles from Step 2 by the total volume from Step 3. Multiply this result by 1000 to find the osmolarity of the mixture in milliosmoles per liter.

$$562.5\overline{)143.25} = 0.255$$

$$0.255 \times 1000 = 255$$

Total osmolarity of admixture = 255 mOsm/L

FLOW RATES

Intravenous fluids are given to patients for many reasons such as dietary replacement and hydration. As a pharmacy technician, you'll never be responsible for administering these fluids.

But, you may be responsible for calculating the flow rate. The flow rate is the number of milliliters of fluid to administer over one hour (it may also refer to the number of milliliters of fluid to administer per minute).

In order to understand how to calculate the flow rate you must:

- be familiar with the IV fluids
- understand the process of administration
- recognize the type of equipment used

Types of IV Fluids

There are several types of IV fluids. The most commonly used are:

- NS—normal saline 0.9%
- ½NS—normal saline 0.45%
- D5W—dextrose 5% in water
- LR, RL, RLS—lactated Ringer's solution, or Ringer's lactated solution
- D5NS—5% dextrose in normal saline
- D5 ½NS—5% dextrose in 0.45% normal saline

Administration of Intravenous Fluids

IV fluids may be given in small or large volumes. They may be given continuously over a long or short period. Or, they may be given irregularly depending on the patient's needs and physician's orders.

Sometimes, a small-volume bag (minibag) may be piggybacked into the line of a large volume IV. When piggybacking is done manually, the flow rate is measured in drops (gtt) per minute. Special tubing regulates the desired flow rate.

When the flow is done automatically, an **infusion pump** is used. An infusion pump is an automatic device used with an IV system for delivering medication at regular intervals in specific quantities.

The pump infuses, or delivers, medication into the IV line according to a preset program. This is much easier than having to administer medication manually at certain intervals round the clock.

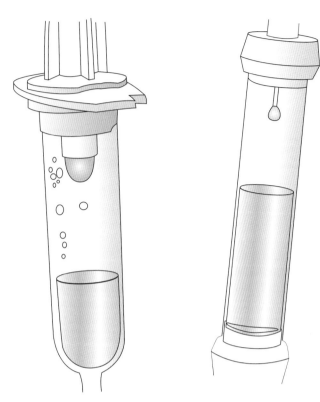

FIGURE 3-1 IV Drip Chambers: Macrodrip (left) and Microdrip (right).

Intravenous Administration Sets for Manual Infusion

IV fluids that are administered manually use infusions sets. Infusion sets consist of plastic tubing attached to one end of an IV bag and at the other end a needle or catheter inserted into a blood vessel. There are two basic types of infusion sets (Fig. 3-1):

- microdrip
- macrodrip

Microdrip Infusion Sets

To deliver 1 mL of fluid to the patient, 60 drops must fall (60 gtt = 1 mL). Microdrip infusion sets always deliver 60 drops of fluid per minute (gtt/mL).

Macrodrip Infusion Sets

Macrodrip amounts per milliliter differ according to the manufacturer. For example, macrodrip sets from Baxter deliver 10 gtt/mL; Abbot sets deliver 15 gtts/mL. The package label or insert will always indicate the drops per milliliter. This information is essential in determining the flow rate of an IV infusion.

Calculating Intravenous Flow Rates

When IV medication is delivered by infusion pump, the flow rate is expressed as milliliters per hour. Also remember that flow rates are always given as whole numbers.

Follow these steps to calculate the flow rate of an IV infusion.

Step 1: *Start with what you know.*
When determining the flow rate, you need a certain amount of required information:

- type of fluid
- volume of fluid
- time period in which you want the IV to flow

Step 2: *Convert.*
Check to see which units need converting. You may need to use **dimensional analysis** to convert them to the units you want. Dimensional analysis is a problem-solving method in which any number or expression can be multiplied by one without changing its value. Or, you might have to apply the principles of ratio and proportion.

Step 3: *Divide.*
When you have the correct units, divide to get the flow rate. Make sure to round up to a whole number if the flow rate is a decimal.

SAMPLE CALCULATIONS

IV Flow Rate

Example 1

Suppose a physician's order is for 100 mL of NS to infuse over 8 hours. What is the flow rate?

Step 1. *Start with what you know.*
Record what you know on the left, and what you don't know on the right.

$$\frac{100mL}{8hours} \longrightarrow X\frac{mL}{hour}$$

Step 2: *No conversion or dimensional analysis is needed since you already have the correct units (mL/hr).*

Step 3. *Divide.*
Simply divide 100 mL by 8 hours to get the flow rate of milliliters per hour.

$$\frac{100}{8} = 12.5 = \frac{mL}{hour}$$

Example 2

Calculate the drop per minute rate needed to deliver cefazolin 500 mg in 50 mL over 15 minutes using a 15-gtt/mL IV set. Calculate rate in drops per minute.

Step 1. *Set up a proportion.*
First, we need to find the number of milliliters per minute, so we set up the following proportion:

$$\frac{50mL}{15min} = \frac{XmL}{1min}$$

Step 2: *Solve the proportion for X.*

$$X = \frac{50}{15} = 3.33\,mL/min$$

Step 3: *Convert.*

Convert mL/min to gtts/min.
Cancel out the units to get the rate in gtts/min.

$$\frac{3.33mL}{1min} \longrightarrow \frac{15gtt}{1mL} = 50\frac{gtt}{min}$$

Therefore, the drip rate needed to deliver 50 mL over 15 minutes using 15-gtt/mL tubing is 50 gtt/min.

CHAPTER HIGHLIGHTS

- The concentration of a CSP based on a medication order can be calculated by setting up a problem as follows: CSP strength (mg/mL) multiplied by a conversion factor (1000 mL/L).
- The correct dose of a CSP can be calculated using the strength of the available stock medication and the prescribed dose.
- The correct dose of a CSP can be calculated using a nomogram to find the patient's BSA.
- A fractional saline CSP is prepared by calculating the amounts needed of the available concentrated saline solution and the concentration of the desired solution.
- The volume of diluent and/or powder in a reconstituted product can be calculated using the final total volume and concentration desired, and the initial volume and concentration of the powder and diluent.
- The alligation method is used to determine the amount of the two products needed to make a final CSP.
- The osmolarity of a solution is calculated by dividing the total milliosmoles of the solution by the total volume (mL) of the solution.
- The flow rate of an IV solution is calculated by dividing the total volume of the fluid by the total delivery time.

QUICK QUIZ

Answer the following multiple-choice questions.

1. What is the concentration in mg/mL of cefazolin 500 mg in 100 mL of D5W?
   a. 5 mg/mL
   b. 50 mg/mL
   c. 500 mg/mL
   d. 5000 mg/mL

2. The Physician orders 250 mg of ampicillin IM. You have a 4 gram vial. The product has been reconstituted to 100 mg/mL. How many milliliters will need to be administered?
   a. 1 ml
   b. 2.5 ml
   c. 4 ml
   d. 5 ml

3. Which of the following is NOT a common diluent?
   a. sterile water
   b. potassium chloride
   c. sodium chloride
   d. heparin

4. You have 70% IPA and water. You need to make 120 mL of 50% vol/vol IPA. Using the alligation method, how many total parts will you have?
   a. 0
   b. 20
   c. 50
   d. 70

5. What is the flow rate of 1 L of NS to run over 8 hours using tubing calibrated to deliver 10 gtt/mL?
   a. 1 gtt/min
   b. 8 gtt/min
   c. 21 gtt/min
   d. 28 gtt/min

Please answer each of the following questions in one to three sentences.

1. Explain the difference between a loading dose and a maintenance dose.

2. How are osmolality and osmolarity measured?

3. What is the purpose of alligation?

4. Calculate the flow rate for the following order: A physician orders 1 L of NS to infuse over 20 hours.

5. What are the ingredients in the following solutions: D5W and D5 ½NS?

Label the following statements as either true or false.

1. ____ The BSA is used when the dosage depends on the patient's weight and height.

2. ____ Maintenance doses are usually larger than loading doses.
3. ____ A nomogram should not be used to determine the body surface area of a child.
4. ____ The concentration of a reconstituted suspension contains 0.75 mg of powder per mL. The final volume of 10 mL contains 7.5 mg of powder.
5. ____ Microdrip amounts per milliliter differ according to the manufacturer.

Match the term in the left column with the correct description from the right column.

1. D5W   a. drops per minute
2. NS   b. process in which a powder is dissolved
3. gtt/min   c. dextrose 5% and water
4. reconstitution d. isopropyl alcohol
5. IPA   e. normal saline

CHAPTER 4

Delivery Systems Equipment

CHAPTER OBJECTIVES

- Identify the different parts of a syringe.
- Identify the different types of syringes available and their unique characteristics.
- Select the appropriate syringe to measure a given volume based on the syringe's calibrations.
- Identify the different parts of the needle.
- Describe filter needles, filter straws, and vented needles.
- Identify when a filter needle or filter straw is used.
- Identify when a vented needle is used.
- Describe the filters used to sterilize products.
- Explain the advantages of a needleless system.
- Explain the difference between large-volume parenterals and piggybacks.
- Compare the advantages and disadvantages of glass bottles versus plastic bags.
- Explain the characteristics of a single-dose vial and a multiple-dose vial.
- Describe the advantages and disadvantages of vials and ampules.
- Explain HEPA filtration.
- Compare and contrast the use of laminar airflow workbenches (LAFWs), biological safety cabinets (BSCs), and compounding aseptic isolators.
- Describe the proper cleaning procedures for an airflow hood.

KEY TERMS

ampule—a sealed glass container that contains a single dose of medication

bevel—the slanted, pointed tip of a needle

biological safety cabinet (BSC)—a vertical flow hood that uses HEPA-filtered air that flows vertically (from the top of the hood towards the work surface) to provide an aseptic work area

calibrations—graduated markings on the outside of a syringe barrel

catheter—a tiny delivery or drainage tube inserted into a vein, artery, or body cavity

critical surface—any surface that comes into contact with a sterile product, container, or closure

delivery system—the pieces of equipment that allow a drug to follow a designated route of administration into the body

filter needle—a needle with a filter molded into the hub designed for one-time use only; used to remove glass particles from a solution

filter straws—thin, sterile straws with a filter molded into the hub; used to draw fluid from an ampule

gauge—the diameter of the opening of a needle, or the lumen

HEPA filter—a high-efficiency particulate air filter used in all aseptic processing areas

hypodermic needle—a needle that fits on the end of a syringe used to inject fluids into or withdraw fluids out of the body

intravenous piggybacks (IVPBs)—IV bags that are administered on a set schedule

laminar airflow workbench (LAFW)—a workbench that uses HEPA-filtered air that flows horizontally (from the back of the bench towards you) to provide an aseptic work area

lumen—the hollow part of a needle

vented needle—a needle with side openings used to reconstitute powdered medication

As a pharmacy technician, you'll frequently handle equipment used in the delivery, preparation, and storage of CSPs. In addition to supplies, there are standard pieces of equipment to assist you in creating a sterile product. It's important to know what these provisions are used for, how to use them properly, and how to keep them sterile. Although the equipment may differ based on the facility, there are universal processes and standards in place to ensure aseptic production.

In this chapter, you will learn how to identify and describe different types of equipment used in delivery systems. These include items such as syringes, needles, vials, ampules, and IV bags. You'll also learn about the different workbench spaces and filtration systems used for CSP preparation.

DELIVERY SYSTEMS

As you know, the pharmacy technician prepares many sterile compounds. Each of these compounds is designed to use a specific route of administration in order to be effective. The pieces of equipment that allow a drug to follow its designated route of administration are referred to as the **delivery system**. In the following sections, you will learn about the equipment used in drug delivery systems.

Syringes

One of the most familiar pieces of a delivery system is a medical syringe. Syringes are made of glass, plastic, or metal. You will most commonly use ones made of plastic. They are used for:

- injection
- irrigation
- withdrawal of fluids

Parts of a Syringe

The parts of a syringe (Fig. 4-1) include:

- tip
- rubber plunger tip
- barrel
- flange
- plunger
- flat knob

All syringes include a hollow barrel with a close-fitting plunger that is attached to one end. A tip designed to connect to a needle, catheter, or other attachment is at the other end of the barrel. Some syringes are designed to have nothing connect to them, such as those used for oral dosing or irrigation.

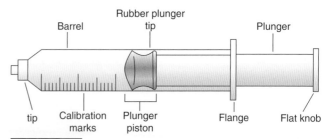

FIGURE 4-1 Various parts of a hypodermic syringe.

When the tip end of the syringe is inserted into a liquid and the plunger is pulled out, the barrel fills with liquid. When the plunger is pushed in, the liquid is forced out through the syringe tip.

Kinds of Syringes

Syringes vary in size from 1 mL (or 1 cc) to 60 mL (or 60 cc). The size used depends on the volume needed.

All hypodermic syringes are marked with calibrations showing milliliters or smaller divisions depending on the size of the syringe.

Two special types of syringes used to administer medications are tuberculin syringes and insulin syringes.

Tuberculin Syringe

Tuberculin (TB) syringes are narrow and have a total capacity of 1mL. Each TB syringe has 100 calibration lines. TB syringes are used for:

- newborn doses
- pediatric doses
- intradermal skin tests
- small doses in adults
- injections just beneath the skin

Insulin Syringe

Insulin syringes are used only for administering insulin to diabetic patients. The insulin syringe has a total capacity of 1 mL, but uses a different calibration system than other syringes.

The 1-mL volume is marked as units (U). The units represent the strength of the insulin per milliliter. Most of the insulin that is used today is U-100, which means that it has 100 units of insulin per milliliter. On the syringe, large lines mark each group of ten units. Five smaller lines divide the ten units into groups of two. Usually, each small line represents two units, but in some syringes it may be one line to one unit.

Syringe Tips

Some syringes are named for the type of tip they have. Here are some you are likely to encounter:

- luer-lock—a syringe tip with a screw-on fitting for the needle; keeps leaks to a minimum

- slip tip—a syringe tip that allows the needle to be easily slipped or pressed on; not as efficient at preventing leaks as the luer-lock
- catheter tip—a long tip, not for injection, but used for cleaning out tissue, for filling body cavities, or for attaching a feeding tube
- eccentric tip—wide syringe tip usually used for oral applications

Critical Surfaces of Syringes

Part of practicing sterile technique is making sure that all **critical surfaces** remain free from contamination. A critical surface is defined as any surface that comes into contact with a sterile product, container, or closure.

Certain parts of a syringe, such as the tip and the plunger are considered critical surfaces. Special care must be taken to assure that these surfaces remain sterile and that the contents inside do not become contaminated. When holding a syringe, you should hold it by the barrel. You can use the flat knob on the end to move the plunger.

In Chapter 2, you learned about the importance of the laminar airflow workbench, or LAFW. In order to preserve the syringe's sterility, you must open the syringe package within the air space of the LAFW.

Some syringes are manufactured with a needle and cap or a protective covering over the tip. If the syringe is packaged with just a protective covering, you must not remove the covering until a needle is ready to be attached. You should complete this process as quickly as possible to avoid contamination.

Syringe Calibrations

Medical syringes have graduated markings on the outside of the barrel. These markings are called **calibrations**, and they differ according to the size and type of syringe. Remember, an insulin syringe is marked in units for measuring insulin and a tuberculin syringe is marked in milliliters up to 1 mL per syringe.

Let's take a look at a few more syringes.

- The 3-mL syringe is marked for each tenth: 1.1 mL, 1.2 mL, 1.3 mL, etc.
- The 5-mL syringes are also marked in tenths, but only reflect every two tenths: 3.2 mL, 3.4 mL, 3.6 mL, etc.
- The 10-mL syringes are also marked in tenths and reflect every two tenths: 3.2 mL, 3.4 mL, 3.6 mL, etc.
- The 20-mL, 30-mL, 50-mL, and 60-mL syringes are marked in whole numbers, or 1-mL increments: 1 mL, 2 mL, 3 mL, etc.

Measuring from the Plunger Tip

Remember, the plunger is the part of the syringe that draws the fluid into the barrel and then pushes it out.

PROCEED WITH CAUTION

Sharps Awareness

Syringes are meant to be used one time only. After use, they should be placed in a plastic puncture-resistant container often called a "sharps container" (Fig. 4-2). Needles are also disposed of in a sharps container. You should *never* force materials into the opening or reach your hand inside the sharps container, so as to avoid needle-stick injuries.

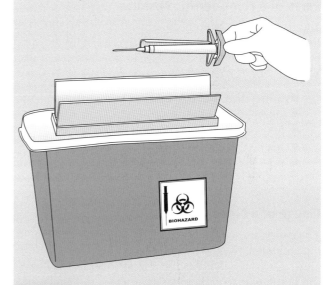

FIGURE 4-2 A sharps container is used for disposal of needles and syringes.

When measuring fluid, you must be alert to which type of tip is on the plunger. Some plunger tips come to a point, while others are flat.

Regardless of the type of tip, you will measure from where the plunger hits the side of the syringe barrel.

Measuring Accurately with a Syringe

Choosing the right syringe for the right amount of fluid is key to using a syringe accurately. For example, you wouldn't want to use a 1-mL tuberculin syringe to draw 2.5 mL of fluid, because you would have to fill it three times. Likewise, you wouldn't use a 30-mL syringe to draw 2 mL of fluid.

When measuring volumes, you'll have to round numbers up or down. Here is a list of rounding suggestions based on syringe volumes:

- 1-mL syringe—accurate to 0.01 mL
- 3-mL syringe—accurate to 0.1 mL
- 5-mL syringe—accurate to 0.2 mL
- 10-mL syringe—accurate to 0.2 mL
- syringes larger than 10 mL—accurate to 1 mL

TIP Until you are comfortable with measuring, you should avoid filling a syringe above 80% of the total volume capacity.

Needles

The **hypodermic needle** is a needle that fits onto the end of a syringe. It's used to inject a specific amount of fluid into, or withdraw a specific amount of fluid out of, the body.

Parts of a Hypodermic Needle

You'll learn that hypodermic needles can be different lengths and different gauges, but they all share the same basic parts. Figure 4-3 shows a diagram and description of these parts.

- hub—the base that attaches to the syringe
- shaft—the longest section
- bevel—the slanted, portion of the needle
- heel—the edge of the bevel closest to the hub
- tip—the end of the needle furthest from the hub

Gauge of a Needle

The **gauge** of a needle refers to the diameter of the opening, or **lumen**. Needle gauges usually range from 28 to 16, although insulin needles are as small as 30 gauge. Here's the tricky part to remember—the *larger* the gauge, the *smaller* the opening. A 30 gauge needle, for example, has a much smaller opening than an 18 gauge needle.

Length of a Needle

Length is another variation of a hypodermic needle. Needle length depends on the route of administration as well as on the body part chosen for injection. Remember from Chapter 2 that a needle may be inserted below the skin, into a vein, or deep into thick muscle tissue.

For example, insulin syringes have a small gauge and a shorter needle. They are used for subcutaneous injections. This helps make daily insulin injections easier and not as painful.

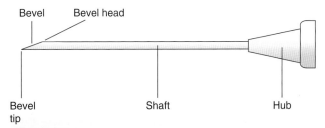

Bevel   Bevel head

Bevel   Shaft   Hub
tip

FIGURE 4-3 Parts of a standard hypodermic needle. (With permission from Thompson, J. E. (2009). *A Practical Guide to Contemporary Pharmacy Practice*. 3rd Ed. Baltimore, MD: Wolters Kluwer Health/Lippincott Williams & Wilkins.)

 PROCEED WITH CAUTION

Filter Needle Use

Only use a filter needle to withdraw from an ampule *or* to inject after withdrawing from an ampule. If you use it both to withdraw and to inject, then the filter particles are injected!

Needles may be anywhere from 3/8 of an inch to 3½ inches, and sometimes longer.

Filters

Filters are often used in combination with needles or other CSP equipment to help prevent or remove contamination. The size of the filter varies according to use. Here are a few common sizes you'll encounter:

- 0.22-micron filter—removes bacteria and particulates
- 0.45-micron filter—removes general particulates
- 1.2-micron filter—removes fungi and particulates
- 5-micron filter—coarse filter; removes glass shards and other particulates

As a pharmacy technician, you'll encounter filter needles, filter straws, and vented needles.

Filter Needles

Filter needles are molded into the hub of the needle and are designed for one-time use only. They remove glass shards that may contaminate a solution when using a glass ampule.

Filter Straws

A **filter straw** is a thin, flexible, sterile straw with a filter in the hub. Filter straws are used to withdraw a single dose of fluid from a sterile glass ampule. Since it's not a needle, it cannot be used to inject.

Vented Needles

Vented needles are used primarily for reconstituting a powdered medication. This type of needle usually has side openings and a thin wall that act as filters to help minimize spraying and foaming during the reconstitution process. You'll learn more about reconstitution in Chapter 7.

NEEDLELESS SYSTEMS

Instead of using a needle and syringe to withdraw a volume of drug from a vial or ampule and injecting it into a bag, these systems allow for the mixing of the drug and the base solution without the use of a needle and syringe. Some of the systems consist of a vial that is attached directly to the IV bag for mixing. Other systems have the drug and base solution in one bag with a barrier in between. The bag is then rolled up to puncture the barrier and mix the two solutions.

INTRAVENOUS SUPPLIES

There are numerous containers and supplies needed for the delivery of sterile products. As a pharmacy technician, it is important for you to be familiar with these. You're likely to use some of them on a daily basis. Here are some you'll learn about:

- IV administration set
- large-volume IV
- intravenous piggybacks (IVPBs)
- intravenous bags and bottles

Intravenous Administration Set

The parts of an IV system that determine the flow rate of the fluid or medication is called the IV administration set. There are two different types of sets:

- vented set—used for containers that have no venting system (IV bottles)
- unvented set—used for containers that have their own venting system or do not require venting (IV bags)

IV administration sets come with various features including ports for infusing secondary medications and filters for blocking microbes.

The tubing also varies. Some types are designed to enhance the proper functioning of devices that help regulate the infusion rate. Other tubing is used specifically for continuous or intermittent infusion or for infusing parenteral nutrition and blood.

There are two main types of IV bags as well:

- large-volume
- intravenous piggybacks (IVPBs)

Large-Volume Intravenous Bags

A large-volume IV bag is sometimes called a large-volume IV drip or a continuous infusion. These are administered continuously and are often used for fluid replacement or for maintenance fluids. A large-volume IV bag usually contains one of the following amounts of fluid:

- 500 mL
- 1 L (1000 mL)

Intravenous Piggybacks

The other type of IV bagging, **intravenous piggybacks (IVPB)**, are administered on a set schedule (e.g., twice a day, three times a day). IVPB bags are generally smaller than large-volume IV bags. This makes sense since they are added on, or "piggybacked," onto a large-volume IV bag.

For example, solutions of antibiotics are often piggybacked onto a large-volume IV bag. A typical IVPB bag contains one of the following amounts of fluid:

- 250 mL
- 100 mL
- 50 mL

Intravenous Bags and Bottles

IV solutions are most commonly prepared in flexible plastic bags, or glass bottles. Both bags and bottles are typically available in five sizes:

- 50 mL
- 100 mL
- 250 mL
- 500 mL
- 1000 mL

The most common type of container used is the flexible IV bag. There are many advantages to using flexible plastic bags over glass bottles. Plastic bags:

- are lighter than glass bottles
- are less expensive than glass bottles
- are easy to see through
- are non-breakable
- take up less volume than plastic or glass bottles

Glass bottles are usually used when the medication is not compatible in a plastic bag due to either absorption or adsorption.

- Absorption—the drug is absorbed into the plastic bag (i.e., nitroglycerin)
- Adsorption—the drug is adsorbed onto the surface of the plastic bag (i.e., insulin)

Both of these result in a loss of drug. Nitroglycerin is typically made in a glass bottle. Insulin, although it is adsorbed, is typically dispensed in plastic with the adsorption taken into account.

DOSAGE CONTAINERS

Medications are supplied from the manufacturer in different types of containers and volumes. Depending on the medication, the manufacturer may package their product in a single-dose vial, multiple-dose vial, or an **ampule**.

Ampules

An ampule is a sealed container made entirely of glass containing a single dose of medication. Once you open an ampule and remove the contents with a filter needle, you must discard the container. Remember, ampules are intended for one-time use only.

When you open an ampule, tiny shards of glass may mix in with the contents. You can extract these unwanted particles by using a filter needle or straw. The filter straw can only be used to withdraw contents from an ampule. The filter needle should only be used one time – to withdraw or to inject. Remember that you must discard the filter needle or straw after using it.

Also, you should always open ampules in an airflow hood using the following procedure:

Single-Dose Vials

Single-dose vials contain one dose of medication and are discarded after one use. For this reason, manufacturers do not add unnecessary preservatives. Preservatives are extremely harmful in situations such as the following:

- pediatric dilutions
- epidurals (an injection of anesthesia into the areas surrounding the spinal column)
- intrathecals (an injection of anesthesia into the areas surrounding the spinal column; usually given during birthing process in place of an epidural)

The top of a single-dose vial has a rubber stopper. The needle pierces the stopper in order to draw fluid. You must insert the needle correctly into the stopper (this is known as "coring"). Otherwise, rubber pieces may break off into the solution, causing contamination.

Even though single-dose vials are designed for one time use, they may be reused again for a limited period of time. You must document the date and time of the first puncture in order to use the remaining contents in the vial.

Multiple-Dose Vials

Multiple-dose vials allow you to use the contents more than once. This means that the rubber stopper of a multiple-dose vial is punctured more than once, thereby exposing the contents of the vial to air. Because of this, multiple-dose vials contain preservatives to keep the contents stable.

All vials should be dated and stored according to the manufacturer's requirements. Check stored vials frequently and discard those that are no longer considered stable. Remember that stability is the ability of a CSP to remain effective until used, or until the expiration date has been reached.

T I P You should always check the expiration date on the vial. Also review the information on the package insert. You'll find that you must refrigerate some types of products stored in vials. If you have any doubts about the age or stability, toss it out.

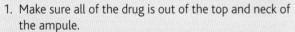

PROCEDURE

Opening Ampules

1. Make sure all of the drug is out of the top and neck of the ampule.
2. Swab the neck of the ampule with IPA.
3. Allow the ampule to dry. Place the head of the ampule between the thumb and index finger on one hand. Hold the body of the ampule by the thumb and index finger of the other hand. You can place a clean swab on the neck of the ampule to prevent cuts and spraying of glass.
4. Open the ampule to the side of the hood away from the HEPA filter.
5. If the ampule has a dot on it, face the dot in the opposite direction as the ampule is being broken.
6. Exert pressure on both thumbs.
7. Push the ampule away from you in a quick snapping motion. The neck of the ampule should break. If it does not, try turning the ampule slightly and repeating these steps.

When you are finished withdrawing the contents from the ampule, discard the glass in an appropriate container.

PROCEDURE

Withdrawing from vials

1. Swab the rubber stopper with IPA and allow to dry.
2. Assemble the needle and syringe.
3. Pull the syringe plunger back to an amount equivalent to the volume you need to withdraw.
4. Place the tip of the needle on the rubber stopper at a 45 degree angle.
5. As you begin to enter the vial, turn the needle up to a 90 degree angle and continue into the rubber stopper.
6. Inject the air from the syringe into the vial.
7. Invert the syringe and vial 180 degree in a clockwise motion.
8. Withdraw the appropriate volume from the vial.
9. Make sure the syringe and needle are free of air bubbles.
10. Invert the syringe and vial back to the starting position.
11. Withdraw the needle from the rubber stopper.

TABLE 4-1 Clean Air Classifications

Clean Air Classification	ISO Designation	≥ 0.5 μm particles/m³
100	5	3,520
1,000	6	35,200
10,000	7	352,000
100,000	8	3,520,000

SPECIAL EQUIPMENT FOR STERILE COMPOUNDING

Now you know all about the supplies used in the preparation, storage, and delivery of sterile products. But, you might recall from Chapter 2 that there is special equipment to assist you in making sure these products are made in a sterile setting.

The USP requires that you prepare CSPs in an ISO Class 5 clean air environment. Class numbers are used to describe air quality in a designated area. See Table 4-1 from USP 797.

This type of clean air space is provided by powerful filters and three important pieces of equipment:

■ a laminar airflow workbench (LAFW)
■ a biological safety cabinet (BSC)
■ a compounding aseptic isolator (CAI)

High-Efficiency Particulate Air Filtration

In order to satisfy the USP's guidelines for ISO Class 5 environments, high-efficiency particulate air filters, or **HEPA filters**, are used in all aseptic processing areas. These filters extract any particles larger than 0.5 microns. The filters must be tested and certified every six months.

Laminar Airflow Workbench

Most CSPs are compounded in a **laminar airflow workbench (LAFW)**. The LAFW, also called a horizontal laminar flow hood, is a work area that prefilters large contaminants from the workspace and then uses HEPA-filtered air in a horizontal flow to extract smaller particles (Fig. 4-4). This creates an aseptic work area.

Here's how the LAFW works:

1. Regular room air is pulled through a vent in front or on top of the hood by a standard furnace filter.
2. The air is pushed toward the back of the LAFW.
3. The air passes through a HEPA filter.
4. The HEPA-filtered air is then forced over the work area at 90 ft/min, which effectively sweeps particulate matter away from the product you are compounding.

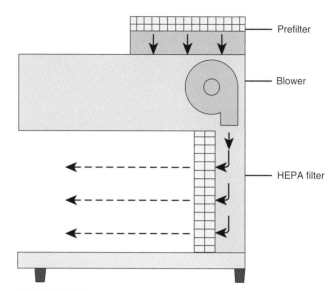

FIGURE 4-4 Horizontal laminar airflow workbench (LAFW). (With permission from Thompson, J. E. (2009). *A Practical Guide to Contemporary Pharmacy Practice*. 3rd Ed. Baltimore, MD: Wolters Kluwer Health/Lippincott Williams & Wilkins.)

Notice that in a LAFW the HEPA-filtered air is blowing directly at you. Anything that you spray while preparing your CSP will blow onto you, which is why hazardous drugs are not prepared in this type of hood.

Biological Safety Cabinet

Unlike the LAFW described above, some hoods blow HEPA-filtered air vertically downward through a top hood and into grills located along the front and back edges of the work surface area. This kind of vertical flow hood is known as a **biological safety cabinet (BSC)**.

These types of hoods can be used for any product preparation, but you're required to use a BSC when working with hazardous compounds such as products used in chemotherapy treatment.

BSCs also have a clear glass or plastic shield that extends partially down the front of the hood. This shield and the vertical flow of air protect you from contamination by drugs processed within.

Compounding Aseptic Isolator

A **compounding aseptic isolator** is a LAFW that is completely enclosed. You can only access the work surface through glove box-type openings. Materials and supplies for aseptic processing enter through special airlock boxes attached to the unit. As with LAFWs and BSCs, this device also uses a HEPA filter system.

Cleaning the Hood

Though you can't see it, some contamination is expected to be present on all types of flow hoods—especially

PROCEDURE

Cleaning the LAFW

1. Start the procedure by removing all jewelry and makeup.
2. Wash hands and forearms with antibacterial soap.
3. Put on a clean, low-shedding gown, hair cover, shoe covers, and mask.
4. Put on sterile protective gloves.
5. Begin the cleaning process by washing the hood walls and surface with sterile water to remove larger particles and those that are water-soluble. Use the following steps:
   ■ Wipe the pole first and any hangers that are attached
   ■ Wipe the sides in a top to bottom, back to front motion using overlapping strokes
   ■ Wipe the work surface from back to front using overlapping strokes
6. Then, use only lint-free material, such as gauze or specially designed wipes, to wipe the LAFW with sterile 70% isopropyl alcohol following the same steps as with the water.
7. When finished, document that you have cleaned the hood.

between product preparations. Therefore, it is critically important to follow a standard procedure for cleaning airflow hoods. Proper cleaning will reduce the risk of cross-contamination of products.

TIP You should clean the entire hood at the beginning and end of every shift. It should also be cleaned after each spill. It is recommended that the surface be cleaned before and after each product or batch of similar products are prepared. Always remember to document each hood cleaning.

CHAPTER HIGHLIGHTS

- The different parts of a syringe are the tip, rubber plunger tip, barrel, flange, plunger, and flat knob.
- Syringes are made of glass, plastic, and/or metal, and they are used for injection, irrigation, withdrawal of fluids, or other parenteral delivery.
- General use syringes come in various sizes and can be used for large or small amounts of fluid.

- Syringes commonly used are the luer-lock and the slip-tip syringe.
- Small syringes, such as insulin syringes and tuberculin syringes, are used to give injections just beneath the skin. An insulin syringe is marked in units, for measuring insulin. A tuberculin syringe is marked in milliliters up to 1 mL per syringe. Larger syringes can be calibrated in increments of 1.0 mL, 0.1 mL, or 0.2 mL.
- The gauge of the needle is the diameter of the opening of needle. Most commonly, needle length may be anywhere from 3/8 inches to 3½ inches.
- The different parts of the needle are the bevel, bevel tip, bevel heel, shaft, and hub.
- Different types of needles include filter needles, filter straws, and vented needles.
- A filter needle is used to extract glass shards from an ampule.
- A filter straw is used to withdraw a single dose of fluid from an ampule.
- A vented needle is used for reconstituting a powdered medication.
- Large-volume parenterals consist of IV bags or bottles of 500 mL or more. Piggybacks consist of IV bags with volumes up to 250 mL.
- Glass IV bottles are more transparent than plastic bags and cannot be poked or pierced. Plastic IV bags take up less space, are less expensive, and lighter.
- Vials are convenient CSP containers. They have a rubber stopper, which is pierced by the needle when drawing up specific amounts of fluid.
- Ampules have glass necks that are snapped off before fluid is drawn.
- There is a risk of rubber contamination when using vials and of glass shard contamination when using ampules.
- HEPA filtration is a powerful filter system used in all CSP workbench spaces. The HEPA filtration system complies with the USP's requirements for an ISO Class 5 environment.
- Laminar airflow workbenches, biological safety cabinets, and compounding aseptic isolators are all used for CSP preparation.
- Laminar airflow workbenches (LAFWs) provide a horizontal airflow within the work space.
- Biological safety cabinets (BSCs) provide a vertical airflow within the workspace.
- Compounding aseptic isolators provide HEPA-filtered air that is completely enclosed.
- Flow hoods should be cleaned regularly and documented. A standard procedure must be followed to avoid contamination.

QUICK QUIZ

Answer the following multiple-choice questions.

1. A filter straw is used to
   a. extract fluids from a vial.
   b. reconstitute a powder.
   c. dilute a solution.
   d. extract shards of glass from an ampule.
2. Which part of the syringe should not be touched?
   a. the barrel
   b. the lip
   c. collar
   d. the plunger
3. A vertical flow hood is also known as a
   a. aseptic isolator.
   b. ISO Class 5 environment
   c. laminar airflow workbench.
   d. biological safety cabinet.
4. A tuberculin syringe is used for all of the following EXCEPT:
   a. pediatric doses.
   b. skin testing.
   c. an insulin injection.
   d. an injection just below the skin.
5. The greatest risk of contamination when using an ampule is from
   a. bits of rubber.
   b. glass shards.
   c. particles of fiber.
   d. flakes of skin.

Please answer each of the following questions in one to three sentences.

1. What are the calibrations on a syringe? What are they used for?

2. Describe how the gauge of a needle is measured. Why would a certain gauge be used instead of another?

3. Compare and contrast multiple-dose vials with single-dose vials.

4. Explain the differences between a luer-lock syringe and a luer-slip syringe.

5. Describe some of the characteristics of the large-volume IV and IV piggybacks. What is the relationship between the two?

Label the following statements as either true or false.

1. _____ A filter needle is used to reconstitute a powder medication.
2. _____ The larger the gauge of a needle, the smaller the opening.
3. _____ A large-volume IV bag contains 500 mL or more of fluid.
4. _____ The surfaces of a LAFW should always be wiped from front to back.
5. _____ HEPA stands for high-efficiency particulate air.

Match the term in the left column with the correct description from the right column.

1. gauge — a. a tiny tube inserted into a vein
2. catheter — b. a sealed glass container
3. ampule — c. the size of the opening of a hypodermic needle
4. intravenous — d. the slanted, pointed tip of a hypodermic needle
5. bevel — e. within a vein

Environment

CHAPTER OBJECTIVES

- Identify the characteristics of a clean room.
- Identify ideal design components for a clean room.
- Explain the differences between the ante-area and buffer area and explain the activities that occur in each.
- Identify the impact of pharmacy staff traffic on airflow patterns.
- Evaluate the differences between positive- and negative-pressure rooms.
- Distinguish the differences between ISO classes 5, 7, and 8.
- Identify and evaluate the standard components of environmental monitoring.
- Explain the purpose and process of particle counting.
- Explain the purpose and process of air and surface sampling.
- Explain the practice of fingertip sampling.
- Describe appropriate cleaning and disinfecting procedures.
- Evaluate proper temperature settings in controlled temperature areas.

KEY TERMS

agar—a gelatinous substance used to collect cultures

ACPH—air changes per hour

ante-area—the vicinity located directly outside the clean room; the first line of air-quality control in a clean room layout

ante room—a room located directly outside the clean room where gowning occurs and compounding supplies are stored

buffer area—the vicinity where the primary engineering control is located and where CSP supplies are prepared

clean room—a room in which the air quality, temperature, and humidity are highly regulated to reduce the risk of cross-contamination

direct compounding area (DCA)—a critical area in the primary engineering control in which critical sites are exposed to unidirectional HEPA-filtered air

laminar flow—air flow that moves in parallel from ceiling to floor or from wall to wall with uniform velocity and minimal turbulence

negative-pressure room—an area in which the air pressure is lower than in nearby spaces so that air flows into the room

positive-pressure room—an area in which the air pressure is higher than the air pressure in nearby vicinities so that the air flows out of the room

primary engineering control (PEC)—the equipment that provides an ISO Class 5 environment for the exposure of critical sites when compounding sterile preparations; LAFW, BSC, CAI

As you've learned, it's only recently that the USP created a set of enforceable sterile compounding standards that are widely available and accepted. These standards provide the procedures and requirements that apply to the environment in which you prepare CSPs. As a pharmacy technician, it's vital to know your environment and the standards to make it safe and sterile.

In this chapter, you'll discover how these standards are applied in establishing a clean room environment for preparing sterile products. You'll identify three primary areas in a clean room and how the presence of pharmacy staff affects airflow patterns. You'll also be able to apply the appropriate ISO classes of air quality required in different areas in a compounding facility. Finally, you'll learn about the procedures involved in environmental monitoring.

CLEAN ROOM

To prepare sterile products, you must start with a clean environment. This environment is referred to as a **clean room** (Fig. 5-1). A clean room is an area in which the air quality, temperature, and humidity are highly regulated to reduce the risk of cross-contamination. Here are some of the initial requirements for a clean room:

- air quality that meets the International Organization for Standardization (ISO) class standards
- HEPA-filtered air
- access to only those personnel who are trained and authorized to perform sterile compounding and facility cleaning

Clean Class Standards

The ISO has created a specific set of standards to maintain a safe and clean environment. The classifications are broken down into the maximum number of allowable particles per room. This number depends on the type of work performed in that area.

If the standards permit a greater number of particles, the air-quality requirements are less rigid and the

class number increases. For example, an area that must meet ISO Class 5 standards will have more particles in the air than a ISO Class 3 area.

There are three classes that are important in preparing CSPs and you'll learn about them in this chapter:

- ISO Class 5
- ISO Class 7
- ISO Class 8

ISO Class 5

You'll need ISO Class 5 air quality when your work involves critical sites. Remember, a critical site is any location in which contaminants might come into contact with a CSP. Fluid pathways, such as injection ports, or openings, such as needle hubs or opened ampules, are common examples of critical sites.

An excellent example of where you'll encounter an ISO Class 5 environment is the **primary engineering control** (PEC). The PEC is the equipment that provides an ISO Class 5 environment for the exposure of critical sites when compounding sterile preparations.

You'll find LAFWs, compounding aseptic isolators (CAIs), and BSCs—the equipment you learned about in Chapter 4—are all PECs.

ISO Class 7

An ISO Class 7 environment includes the main compounding area. The clean room and **buffer area**— the room where the PEC is located and where CSP supplies are prepared—are examples of ISO Class 7 environments. In an ISO Class 7 environment, you'll:

- stage compounding components and supplies
- prepare CSPs inside a LAFW, BSC or CAI

When preparing hazardous drugs, the ante room – a separate room you enter prior to entering the clean room – is an ISO Class 7 environment.

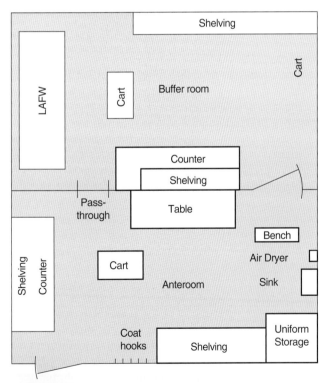

FIGURE 5-1 Example of a clean room and ante area floor plan. Note locations of the anteroom, buffer area, and LAFW. (With permission from Thompson, J. E. (2009). *A Practical Guide to Contemporary Pharmacy Practice*. 3rd Ed. Baltimore, MD: Wolters Kluwer Health/Lippincott Williams & Wilkins.)

 PROCEED WITH CAUTION

Critical Information

Contamination is more likely to occur when there are more exposed areas of critical sites. Airborne contaminants, especially those shed from pharmacy staff members, are more likely to reach critical sites than contaminants that are stuck to the floor or below the workspace level.

Because of the greater risk of contamination, you'll only work with critical sites in an environment meeting or exceeding ISO Class 5 standards.

ISO Class 8

An ISO Class 8 environment is a transition area. It's the vicinity of the clean room that will have the highest number of particles in the air.

The **ante-area** for nonhazardous drugs is an example of an ISO Class 8 environment. The ante-area is the vicinity located directly outside the clean room. This area is the first line of air-quality control in a clean room layout.

Layout

The layout of the clean room is based on the main types of CSPs that the staff will handle in that facility. There are two main types of layouts considered starting points when designing a clean room:

- 12-hour or less beyond-use date (BUD) layout (remember, you determine the BUD by the date or time after which you can no longer store or transport a product)
- low-, medium-, or high-risk CSPs layout

These main designs are arranged differently, but you can think of both in terms of a bull's-eye. The quality of air increases as you move toward the **direct compounding area (DCA)**. The DCA is a critical area in the PEC in which critical sites are exposed to unidirectional HEPA-filtered air. You can think of the DCA as the center of the bull's-eye.

12-Hour or Less BUD Layout

According to a 12-hour or less BUD layout, the most critical operation area is placed in the PEC in a segregated compounding area. As long as other criteria are met, these CSPs do not have to be prepared in an ISO Class 7 clean room. The following criteria for the environment must be met:

- Products must be prepared in an ISO Class 5 PEC.
- The segregated compounded area cannot contain any unsealed windows or doors that open to the outside.
- It must not be a high traffic area.
- Personnel must wash their hands and garb just like in a clean room.

Compounding personnel should recognize that the lack of an ISO Class 7 clean room increases the chance of contamination. Proper technique, handwashing, garbing, cleaning and other activities that will decrease the likelihood of contamination are essential.

Low-, Medium-, or High-Risk Layout

A facility set up to prepare CSPs may be considered to have low-, medium-, or high-risk levels within its layout.

The quality of the air increases as you move from the outer boundaries toward the DCA. In this type of setting, the compounding facility ensures that the ISO Class 5 environment is properly arranged to accommodate each risk level. As a pharmacy technician, you're responsible for determining the risk level of the CSP you're compounding. Once you determine the risk level, you'll know where you'll work in the clean room. You'll learn more about determining risk levels in Chapter 7.

The placement of devices or objects that are not essential to compounding in this area should be restricted or limited. Some of these items are:

- printers
- computers
- carts
- cabinets or other storage containers

Ante-Area

The ante-area is the outermost region in the clean room layout. The ante-area is the location where you'll do high-particulate–generating activities such as:

- washing your hands
- dressing in proper garb
- staging components

The ante-area is also a transition area where:

- air flows from clean to dirty areas, thereby maintaining constant air pressure relationships
- heating, ventilating, and air-conditioning (HVAC) is kept to a minimum

Anteroom

Hazardous drugs are prepared in a room similar to the low-, medium-, and high-risk products. However, hazardous drugs must have an adjacent anteroom instead of an ante area. And, the anteroom must meet ISO Class 7 standards instead of ISO Class 8.

A separate, walled room with positive pressure will ensure that contaminants are not introduced into other areas.

Buffer Area

The buffer area is the area inside the clean room where the PEC is located. Here you'll prepare the supplies you use when compounding products. The buffer area is segregated by HEPA-filtered air to reduce the likelihood of cross-contamination.

The amount of HEPA-filtered air required depends on:

- the number of pharmacy staff working in the room
- the type of compounding performed
- the temperature of the area in that part of the clean room

It's important that the PEC is located in the buffer area in such a way that it's not in the path of:

- strong air currents from open doors
- air streams from the HVAC
- operator movement in the workspace
- pharmacy staff traffic

Pressure

Air pressure, both positive and negative, plays a significant role in maintaining the air quality in a clean room. Air pressure helps keep drafts from carrying contaminants from one area to another. It also helps stabilize the vapor pressures of hazardous drugs that can become volatile if you don't store them properly.

Positive-Pressure Rooms

A **positive-pressure room** is an area in which the air pressure is higher than the air pressure in nearby vicinities. This ensures that the air flows out of the room. Rooms close to areas that you'll use for high-risk compounding require positive pressure to keep high-risk contaminants from seeping into the workspace.

Negative-Pressure Rooms

A **negative-pressure room** is an area in which the air pressure is lower than in nearby vicinities, so that air flows into the room. Hazardous materials are contained in a negative-pressure room because of their volatile nature. A Compounding Aseptic Containment Isolator (CACI), which is used to handle these volatile materials, is also located in this area.

In a negative-pressure room, it's important that the ventilation system is adequate to change the air on a regular basis. You'll learn more about the process of air changing later in this chapter.

Design

USP Chapter 797 lists specific design requirements for a clean room. The standards allow only furniture, equipment, and supplies necessary to compound in the buffer area. These items must be:

- nonporous
- nonshedding
- impervious to disinfectants

Everything is cleaned and disinfected before it enters the buffer area. Nothing should be removed from the area except to perform the following activities:

- cleaning
- servicing
- calibrating

Surfaces

It's important that the surfaces in the clean room are nonporous, free from cracks, and nonshedding. This assures that there are no spaces on which microorganisms and contaminants can accumulate. These surfaces include:

- ceilings
- walls
- floors
- fixtures
- shelving
- counters
- cabinets

Ceilings, Walls, and Floors

Some clean room ceilings are composed of inlaid panels saturated with a polymer so that they're nonporous and resistant to moisture. The perimeter of each panel is caulked to seal them to the support frame.

Walls are constructed of a flexible material such as a heavy-gauge polymer. The polymer panels are locked together and then tightly sealed. Another option is epoxy-coated gypsum board. When it isn't coated with epoxy, gypsum board is also known as dry wall. This allows the walls to be washed or cleaned regularly.

Floors should be overlaid with wide-sheet vinyl that has heat-welded seams and molding. Since floors are particularly susceptible to settling particles, it is critical that there are no crevices in which contaminants might settle.

Lighting and Work Space

Proper lighting and work space is essential, but both can be troublesome when planning a clean room. Any overhangs, such as windowsills, ledges, and ceiling-level utility pipes, are avoided. Ceiling lighting fixtures must be smooth and sealed tightly to the ceiling.

Work surfaces are made of smooth, nonporous materials. Some of these are:

- stainless steel
- nonporous, molded plastic
- sheet metal

When you're transporting CSPs, a cart with cleanable casters is a useful addition and should be made out of one of the materials listed above.

In addition, there should not be any water sources, such as sinks or floor drains, in the buffer area because these can harbor microorganisms.

HEPA Filtration

HEPA filters in the PEC control airborne contamination. The airflow in the PEC is unidirectional, or a **laminar flow**. This type of flow moves in parallel from ceiling to floor or from wall to wall with uniform velocity and a minimum of turbulence.

Because of the HEPA filter's efficiency at collecting particles, the first air at the face of the filter is free from airborne contamination.

Air Changes

Air-change requirements, measured as air changes per hour (**ACPH**), will maintain the ISO classification standards for each boundary in the clean room. There are several factors that determine the number of ACPH in each area, including:

- the number of pharmacy staff working in the room
- the type of compounding process in use
- the temperature

An ISO Class 7 ante-area or buffer area receiving HEPA-filtered air will receive 30 ACPH or more. The PEC will generate some air changes, but it can't be the sole source of HEPA-filtered air. These areas may have an ISO Class 5 recirculating device. If so, a minimum of 15 ACPH is required as long as the combined ACPH (i.e., from the PEC and from the HVAC system) is not less than 30 ACPH.

Air Flow

HEPA-filtered supply air enters an area at the ceiling level, not at the floor. Return vents into the system are placed on the wall near the floor. This creates a top-down flow of HEPA-filtered air.

The principle of "displacement airflow" is used between buffer and ante-areas. This concept uses low-pressure and an air velocity of 40 feet/minute or more from the buffer area across the line of demarcation that separates the buffer area from the ante area.

Displacement airflow is not appropriate for high-risk compounding, but for low- and medium-risk compounding only.

T I P Because the flow of air is so critical to maintaining the proper ISO class in a clean room, it's necessary that ventilation returns and your equipment does not block registers. You should regularly inspect each register to ensure that air is flowing freely.

ENVIRONMENTAL MONITORING

Now that you've learned what's involved in constructing a clean room, environmental monitoring is what you and facility operators can do to maintain it.

Environmental monitoring guarantees that the clean room is functioning according to standards with low levels of particles. The areas under inspection for this evaluation include:

- ISO Class 5 PECs (LAFW, CAI)
- buffer areas
- ante-areas
- segregated compounding areas

Some of the processes involved in monitoring a clean room are:

- particle counting
- air sampling
- surface sampling
- gloved fingertip sampling
- cleaning and disinfecting
- maintaining set temperatures

Particle Counting

Particle counting involves obtaining samples of non-living airborne particles. Special equipment is used to ensure that the following criteria are met:

- ISO Class 5—no more than 3,520 particles (0.5 micrometers and larger) per cubic meter of air for LAFWs, BSCs, and CAIs
- ISO Class 7—no more than 352,000 particles (0.5 micrometers and larger) per cubic meter of air for any buffer area
- ISO Class 8—no more than 3,520,000 particles (0.5 micrometers and larger) per cubic meter of air for any ante-area

Each facility is responsible for developing a plan of when to conduct particle counts. It is important that counts occur during times of activity instead of only when the area is empty of personnel. The results must be kept on file and made available to regulatory agencies, such as the Joint Commission or the state Board of Pharmacy, upon request.

Particle counts are conducted at these times at a minimum:

- at least every six months
- when the PEC has been relocated
- when the environment has been altered

Air Sampling

Air sampling involves obtaining samples of living airborne particles in ISO Class 5, 7, and 8 environments. Samples are also taken from segregated compounding areas that are at high risk for contamination, including:

- work areas near the ISO Class 5 environment
- counters near doorways
- pass-through areas

Like particle counts, the facility must have a plan of when air sampling must occur. Air samples are taken at the following times at a minimum:

- when equipment or facilities are built
- after equipment or facilities are serviced
- every six months as part of recertification
- in response to end-product concerns

A sampling plan based on the risk involved with the tasks technicians perform in that area must be created. The plan should include:

- location of the sample
- method of collection
- frequency of sampling
- volume of air sampled
- time of day

Air-Sampling Devices

There are many different types of air-sampling equipment. Two common sampling devices are:

- high-sensitivity particle counters
- low-sensitivity counters

These machines are sometimes very large, or some can be small enough to hold in your hand.

An adequate sample is collected faster with a high-sensitivity particle counter than with a low-sensitivity counter. Also, samples are collected easier in dirty rooms compared with cleaner rooms.

Surface Sampling

You learned in Chapter 2 that touch contamination is one of the most common ways that microbes are spread in a compounding area. The practice of surface sampling helps maintain a controlled environment for compounding CSPs. It's useful for evaluating both pharmacy staff procedures and work practices in a compounding facility.

Surface sampling is not as complicated as air sampling and does not require special equipment. Surface collection is performed at the end of compounding,

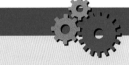

PROCEDURE

Air-Sampling

Here's how the air-sampling process works:

1. The facility creates a sampling plan.
2. 400 to 1,000 liters of air is collected using an air sampler.
3. Slides called microbial growth media plates are prepared.
4. The plates are incubated for a set amount of time.
5. The plates are removed from incubation, and the microorganisms on each plate are counted.
6. The microorganisms are recorded in measurements called colony-forming units (CFU).
7. Steps are taken to determine the source of the microbes, particularly if the organisms are highly pathogenic.

or at regular intervals according to the policies of the facility.

Contact plates and swabs are used in collection. Contact plates are best for sampling regular or flat surfaces. Swabs are best for sampling irregular surfaces, such as equipment.

Contact Plate Collection

A contact plate is covered in a thick layer of **agar**, a gelatinous substance used to collect cultures. The plate is rolled gently across the sampling area. The agar surface will collect any present microbes. The microbes are counted and reported as CFU.

T I P The contact plate will leave a residue after a sample is taken. It's important to thoroughly wipe the surface afterward with a nonshedding wipe soaked in sterile 70% isopropyl alcohol. Alcohol disinfects in the drying process as it evaporates. This process is known as desiccation.

Swab Collection

For swab collection, a swab is gently wiped across the sampling area and planted on agar. As with contact plate collection, the results are reported as CFU.

The sampling data are collected and reviewed regularly to evaluate the control of the environment. Appropriate action is based on resulting CFU counts.

T I P Sterile gloves are the last item you'll put on when dressing to work in a clean room. But your gloves can still be contaminated when they come into contact with nonsterile surfaces during compounding activities. You can disinfect your gloves by rubbing them with sterile 70% IPA. You should do this throughout the compounding process, especially whenever you touch nonsterile surfaces, such as vials, countertops, chairs, and carts. Always allow your gloved hands to dry completely before working.

Gloved Fingertip Sampling

Before you're permitted to compound CSPs, you'll have to complete a "competency evaluation" at least three times when you start working in a facility's clean room. The evaluation involves a gloved fingertip or thumb sampling used to detect any potential microbes.

After you put on the proper safety garments and sterile gloves, you'll press each finger lightly into agar, a gelatinous substance used to collect cultures. Another staff member will put the culture in incubation for a predetermined length of time before it is evaluated. The sample must result in 0 CFU.

If you pass the initial evaluations, future samplings will occur at least once a year. Future gloved fingertip sampling will be conducted immediately after preparing a CSP and before gloves are disinfected with alcohol.

Cleaning and Disinfecting

When you clean and disinfect the surfaces where you prepare CSPs, you're doing your job of keeping microbial infection to a minimum. The areas in a clean room environment that you'll sanitize are:

- ISO Class 5 compounding areas
- buffer areas
- ante-areas
- segregated compounding areas

The type of disinfectants you'll use depends on several factors. These are:

- microbial activity
- inactivation by organic matter
- type of residue
- shelf life of the products in that area

Here's when you should sanitize your work area:

- at the beginning of each work shift
- before each batch preparation is started
- every 30 minutes during continuous compounding periods
- when there are spills
- when surface contamination is suspected or known

You'll disinfect surfaces in ISO Class 5 areas, such as LAFWs, BSCs, and CAIs more frequently because these are areas in which critical sites are often exposed. You've already learned the process for cleaning these pieces of equipment in Chapter 4. Remember: wipe side surfaces from top to bottom.

For all other work areas and clean room surfaces, cleaning and disinfecting is a three-step process:

1. Remove all items from the area that you're about to clean.
2. Clean surfaces by removing loose residue and residue from spills.
3. Wipe down the surfaces with a residue-free disinfecting agent, such as sterile 70% isopropyl alcohol, and allow them to dry.

The floors and work surfaces should be cleaned daily. Emptied shelving, walls, and ceilings should be cleaned at least monthly.

Since some cleaning and disinfecting, such as mopping, may not be performed by pharmacy personnel, training and education is essential to ensure that it is done properly.

T I P You don't have to use alcohol or highly toxic disinfectants on spaces such as floors and countertops. There are many disinfectants on the market you can use to clean light to moderate soiling, such as bleach. You can also use these products to remove dust and debris from storage sites of compounding ingredients. Just be sure you don't compromise the air quality when cleaning.

Temperature

Temperature is a critical factor to keep in mind when you're compounding. If you don't properly monitor the temperature of the air, you're compromising the sterility, stability, and purity of the product. Specific temperature settings are outlined by the USP in order to maintain a stable compounding facility. These are:

- cold temperature: 2-8°C
- freezing temperature: –25-10°C

It's important that you are aware of the storage temperature for CSPs and all compounding ingredients so that you store the products under the proper conditions. You should monitor a controlled temperature at least once a day.

Temperature in controlled areas should be monitored at least daily and documented. Records must be available for review upon request by regulatory agencies.

Temperature Deviation

Although it's important to store products in the proper conditions, there is a small amount of room for deviation. You can store products designated for a controlled cold temperature (e.g., 2 and 8°C) in an area fluctuating between 0 and 15°C. In fact, the manufacturer may even allow increases in temperature up to 25°C as long as the increases do not extend beyond 24 hours.

You can also store most products labeled for a cool place (e.g., between 8 and 15°C) in a standard refrigerator.

Temperature Limits

The proper room temperature in a compounding facility is 20°C or cooler to minimize particle shedding. You'll store some products in a separate controlled room temperature area (e.g., 20-25°C range). You can deviate slightly from this standard as long as it's no more than 5°C warmer or colder.

The manufacturer may allow room-temperature designated CSPs increases in temperature up to 40°C, as long as the increases do not extend beyond 24 hours.

CHAPTER HIGHLIGHTS

- The clean room, buffer area, ante-area, and direct-compounding area comprise a sterile compounding environment.
- ISO Classes 5, 7, and 8 determine the allowable air quality in a clean room environment.
- A clean room requires standardized walls, floors, shelving, ceilings, and equipment.
- All surfaces in a clean room must be nonporous, nonshedding, and impervious to disinfectants.
- Most equipment and surfaces are made of stainless steel, nonporous, molded plastic, or sheet metal.

- Positive and negative pressure can be used to keep contaminants in or out of an area.
- HEPA filters control airborne contamination.
- Low-, medium-, and high-risk CSPs require different compounding environments.
- PECs lend significant help in establishing a sterile workspace.
- Pharmacy staff members are the greatest potential source of contamination in a compounding facility and must be monitored carefully.
- Particle counting and air and surface sampling are monitoring jobs completed by facility operators.
- Fingertip sampling, disinfecting, and maintaining the temperatures are monitoring responsibilities of the pharmacy technician.
- Disinfecting the workspace is an ongoing and demanding job, but it is important for maintaining sterility and purity.

QUICK QUIZ

Answer the following multiple-choice questions.

1. Which of the following materials would you be least likely to find in a clean room?
   a. stainless steel cart
   b. paper towels
   c. laminar airflow workbench
   d. product containers
2. A common source of ISO Class 5 air quality for exposure of critical sites is a/an
   a. laminar airflow workbench.
   b. HVAC system.
   c. positive-pressure room.
   d. exterior ventilation fan.
3. As you move closer to the direct compounding area in a clean room environment,
   a. a greater number of personnel is involved.
   b. the temperature is kept cooler.
   c. the air is more highly purified.
   d. the area is known as "high risk."
4. When establishing traffic patterns in a clean room, it's best to
   a. minimize traffic in and out of the direct compounding area.
   b. regulate the use of shoe covers in the facility.
   c. use multiple points of entry into the ante-area to keep airflow moving.
   d. assign work stations to discourage wandering in the facility.
5. Why should an ISO Class 5 area be disinfected frequently?
   a. because it's a negative-pressure room
   b. because more personnel work in the area at once
   c. because of the CSP's exposure to critical sites
   d. because of the variety of surfaces in the area

Please answer each of the following questions in one to three sentences.

1. Why is it important for surfaces in a clean room to be resistant to damage?

2. Explain the difference between a negative-pressure and a positive-pressure room.

3. Describe activities that are appropriate for an ISO Class 7 environment, and give an example of this type of area.

4. How does personnel traffic affect the airflow in a work area, and how should it be monitored?

5. Name three factors that determine the number of air changes per hour in an ISO-classified environment.

Label the following statements as either true or false.

1. ____ A controlled temperature area should be monitored every 2 hours.
2. ____ The ante-area is appropriate for personnel hand hygiene.
3. ____ The main purpose of a clean room is to reduce the risk of cross-contamination when compounding.
4. ____ An example of a low-risk product is chemotherapy solutions.
5. ____ A common disinfectant in a compounding facility is sterile 70% isopropyl alcohol.

Match the term in the left column with the correct description from the right column.

1. PEC — a. parallel air flow from floor to ceiling and wall to wall
2. laminar flow — b. a gelatinous substance used to collect cultures
3. DCA — c. provides ISO Class 5 environment for the exposure of critical sites
4. ante-area — d. area where critical sites are exposed to unidirectional HEPA-filtered air
5. agar — e. the first line of air-quality control in a clean room layout

CHAPTER **6**

Basic Aseptic Techniques

CHAPTER OBJECTIVES

- List each component of personnel protective equipment.
- Describe the proper garbing procedure and why it is essential.
- Explain proper hand-washing technique.
- Identify appropriate antimicrobial agents used in hand washing.
- Compare and contrast the different types of gloves available.
- Describe how to remove contaminated gloves.

KEY TERMS

antimicrobial soap—an agent that kills microscopic pathogens such as bacteria and other potentially harmful organisms
chlorohexidene gluconate—an antimicrobial soap used for aseptic hand washing, often abbreviated CHG
Corynebacterium—bacteria found on the skin's surface
garb—all elements of personal protective equipment
personnel protective equipment (PPE)—the various pieces of clothing and gear worn by pharmacy technicians to lower the risk of personal infection and the spread of contamination
scrubs—short-sleeved, full-legged, low-particulate garments that can be sterilized and worn under a gown
Staphylococcus—bacteria found on the skin's surface or the mouth, nose, or throat; transmitted by direct contact

As a pharmacy technician, you may find yourself wearing many of the same garments worn by other health care workers. There's a good reason for this—these products have been proven to lower the risk of personal infection and the spread of contamination. The garments you'll wear are just as important as the work you do. Without them, you're compromising your own health and the sterility and stability of the preparations you're compounding. Following the proper procedures for dressing and washing is equally important.

In this chapter, you'll learn about the function and characteristics of each element of personnel protective equipment. You'll also learn the first steps to basic aseptic techniques involved in sterile compounding including the correct procedures for garbing, hand washing, and gloving.

PERSONNEL PROTECTIVE EQUIPMENT

You'll never enter a clean room before you dress in all elements of your **personnel protective equipment (PPE)**—the various pieces of clothing and gear worn to lower the risk of personal infection and the spread of contamination. You may also hear PPE referred to simply as "**garb**." Your PPE is the first line of defense against contamination. It prevents pathogens, fibers, and particles from transferring from your body to the clean room and CSP you're preparing.

Your PPE includes a variety of items that you'll put on in the order listed below:

1. scrubs
2. shoe covers
3. hair covers
4. beard covers
5. face masks
6. gowns
7. eye shields
8. gloves

You'll take a break from garbing to wash your hands after you put on your face mask. After hand washing, you'll finish putting on your garb. You'll learn more about the procedures for garbing and washing your hands later in the chapter.

Scrubs

Scrubs are short-sleeved, full-legged, low-particulate garments that you can wear under your gown. Sometimes, you're permitted to wear regular clothing under your gown, but most compounding facilities require scrubs.

Shoe Covers

You'll wear disposable covers over your shoes to keep dirt and other particles from polluting the clean room floor. Shoe covers are specially made to be low particulate so their fibers won't contribute to preexisting floor contamination.

> **T I P** As an alternative to shoe covers, you can use a dedicated pair of shoes which you'll store in the ante-area. You should clean them thoroughly on a regular basis. A plastic clog may be appropriate since they could easily be sanitized prior to and after use.

Hair Cover

Hair covers are soft, disposable, low-particulate caps that fit over your head and completely cover your hair. Wearing a hair cover prevents hair and particles from the scalp from contaminating the clean room and CSPs.

Beard Cover

A beard cover is a soft, disposable, low-particulate item that covers a beard, moustache, sideburns, or other facial hair. If you don't have any facial hair, a face mask is sufficient.

Face Mask

A face mask is a low-particulate cover that you'll wear over your mouth and nose. The thin metal strip located in the face mask should be molded over the bridge of your nose to ensure proper fit. You'll be able to breathe easily through it, and it's soft enough that it won't irritate your skin. You should dispose of your face mask every time you leave the clean room.

Gown

You'll put on a protective gown over your regular clothes or scrubs after you wash your hands, but before you enter the buffer area.

A gown is non-shedding and disposable, but sometimes you'll wear it for an entire shift before tossing it out. The sleeves fit snugly around the wrists, and the gown covers all undergarb to prevent particle and fiber shedding. It will either snap, tie, velcro or button in the front or back.

Eye Shield

An eye shield protects your eyes from harmful products that might splatter while compounding. Most shields will comfortably fit over eyeglasses. You'll generally wear an eye shield only when preparing hazardous drugs or when disinfecting a clean room.

You can sterilize most eye shields by placing them in an autoclave, or dispose of them in the proper receptacle.

Gloves

Gloves cover your hands and therefore prevent the transfer of contaminating substances from under fingernails, in scratches, or other creases on your hands. There are various types of gloves available. You'll learn more about these later in the chapter.

GARBING

Your garbing procedure begins in the ante-area before you enter the clean room and before washing your hands. As you have just learned, there are many pieces of PPE that are part of your garb. It might seem like a lot to remember, but with practice, your garbing procedure will become second nature.

The following Procedures describe the recommended step-by-step procedure for dressing in your protective equipment as well as removing it.

PROCEDURE

Garbing (Fig.6-1)

1. Remove cosmetics, jewelry, and outer clothing such as coats, jackets, hats, scarves, and sweaters.
2. Change into scrubs if your facility requires them.
3. Put on dedicated shoes or shoe covers one at a time. As you put these on, be aware of the line of demarcation separating the clean and dirty sides of the ante area. Put the first shoe cover on, and then step with that foot over the line of demarcation to put on the second shoe cover. After putting on the second shoe cover, step over the line of demarcation into the clean side of the ante area.
4. Put on your head cover. Make sure that all of your hair is tucked neatly inside.
5. Put on your beard cover if necessary.
6. Put on your face mask tight enough that there are no side gaps.
7. Wash your hands (as described later in the chapter).
8. Put on your protective gown.
9. Prior to putting gloves on, disinfect hands using a waterless alcohol-based surgical hand scrub with persistent activity. Allow the hands to dry.

10. Put on appropriate gloves (as described later in the chapter). Examine the gloves to make sure there are no defects, tears or holes. Make sure the gloves are of the appropriate size.
11. Enter the buffer area immediately without touching anything on the way.

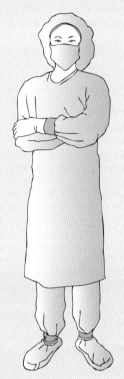

FIGURE 6-1 Pharmacy technician in full protective garb.

PROCEDURE

Removing Your Garb

1. When you are finished compounding, exit the clean room and enter the ante-area.
2. Remove your eye shield and place it in a storage container designated for equipment to be sterilized.
3. Remove shoe covers one at a time and dispose of them in a facility-approved container.
4. Remove your protective gown and dispose of it unless you'll use it again that same day. In this case hang it up in the ante-area by the entrance to the clean room.
5. Remove your mask by holding the top strings. Dispose of the mask by holding it by the ties only. Carefully dispose of the mask.
6. Remove the rest of your garb items and carefully dispose them.

HAND WASHING

A critical step in basic aseptic technique is proper hand washing. You'll do this before you put on your gown and gloves. It sounds simple, but it's more thorough than your everyday wash with liquid soap and warm water.

As you have already learned, bacteria can easily contaminate a CSP. All of the surfaces on your body are covered in bacteria. Careful hand washing removes nearly all microbes commonly found on the hands such as:

■ *Staphylococcus*—bacteria found on the skin's surface or the mouth, nose, or throat; transmitted by direct contact
■ *Corynebacterium*—bacteria found on the skin's surface transmitted by direct contact; a common cause of skin infection or disease

Proper hand washing also removes yeasts.

You'll wash your hands in the ante-area before entering the clean room or compounding area. What to use, how to wash, and how to dry are important factors in aseptic technique.

Products Used for Aseptic Hand Washing

During the hand-washing procedure, you'll use soaps such as Hibiclens, Vionex, or **chlorohexidene gluconate (CHG)**, an antimicrobial soap used for aseptic hand washing. An **antimicrobial soap** kills microscopic pathogens such as bacteria and other potentially harmful organisms.

Proper Hand-Washing Technique

The entire hand washing process should take about two to three minutes. Here are some things you should do before washing your hands:

■ Keep your nails short—no longer than ¼ of an inch beyond the end of the fingertip. Long nails harbor more dirt and microorganisms than short nails.
■ Remove artificial fingernails. These also harbor dirt and microorganisms.
■ Remove your rings and watch. You should have no jewelry on from the elbow to the wrist.
■ Gather the supplies (soap, paper towels, waste container, and nailbrush) you'll need if they are not present in the hand-washing area.

The Procedure below describes how to wash your hands properly.

Because frequent hand washing strips the skin of natural oils, this simple procedure can result in dryness, cracking, and irritation. Dry, cracked skin is more likely to flake and cause particle contamination.

To help minimize irritation, rinse your hands thoroughly, making sure they are free from residue. If you

PROCEDURE

Hand Washing

1. Adjust the water temperature until it's at a comfortable temperature. Adjust the flow to avoid excessive splashing.
2. If using a pre-packaged disinfecting agent, open the package and remove the nail pick. Pick under nails using a nail pick or brush.
3. Wet hands and arms. If using a pre-packaged disinfecting agent, squeeze the sponge to evenly distribute the disinfectant on the sponge.
4. Using a circular motion, clean all four surfaces of each finger.
5. Move to the hand, wrist and arm cleaning all sides with a circular motion. Be careful not to touch the sink, faucet or other objects that might contaminate the hands during the process.
6. Repeat on other arm.
7. Rinse holding hand upright and allowing the water to run from the fingertips down the elbow. Make sure all soap residue has been rinsed.
8. Repeat on other arm.
9. Pat dry from fingertips to elbows using a dry, clean lint-free paper towel. If available, use an electric dryer.
10. Repeat on other arm.
11. Turn off the water with a dry, clean lint-free paper towel. Do not touch the faucet with the bare hand when turning it off. Avoid rubbing, which can cause irritation and generate skin particles.

develop dermatitis—inflammation of the skin—a physician should evaluate you to determine whether you should continue working until the condition resolves.

GLOVING

The gloves you'll use as a pharmacy technician not only help prevent contamination of CSPs, they'll protect any open wounds or scratches on your hands from infection.

PROCEED WITH CAUTION

Moisture Awareness

Microorganisms spread quickly on wet surfaces. Avoid splashing water on yourself or the floor and avoid touching the sink or faucets. They're considered contaminated surfaces. If the sink isn't equipped with knee or foot controls, turn off the faucets by gripping them with a dry, clean lint-free paper towel to avoid recontaminating your hands.

It's essential that you disinfect your gloves with IPA when you enter the clean room. You should also routinely disinfect them throughout the compounding process as you make contact with surfaces.

There is no set procedure for putting gloves on, but taking them off can be tricky if you've spilled hazardous products or a substance you are allergic to on them. In this case, you'll need to make sure you don't contaminate your skin. The following Procedure describes how to safely remove your gloves.

There are several different types of gloves you'll use in a compounding facility:

- sterile or non-sterile
- latex or latex-free
- powdered or non-powdered

Sterile and Non-Sterile Gloves

Sterile gloves are worn when sterile conditions are critical. For example, you'll always wear sterile gloves when compounding preparations or while working inside a flow hood.

Non-sterile gloves are worn when you simply want to protect your hands or prevent the spread of particles. For example, you'll wear non-sterile gloves for activities conducted outside the clean room.

Latex and Latex-Free Gloves

Both sterile and non-sterile gloves may be made of latex. Latex gloves are made from natural rubber. They are comfortable and easy to use when preparing CSPs. Latex gloves are also very elastic, which makes them easy to put on.

An allergy to latex is not an uncommon occurrence. In these cases, gloves are also available in non-latex materials such as:

- polyisoprene
- vinyl
- nitrile rubber

However, non-latex gloves do not have the flexibility or sensitivity of latex gloves. Also, high-grade non-latex gloves, such as nitrile rubber gloves, are expensive; they can cost twice as much as latex gloves.

Powdered and Non-Powered Gloves

Some gloves are powdered on the inside with cornstarch to make them easier to put on and take off. However, cornstarch can inhibit chapped skin from healing and it may cause irritation on cuts or sores on the hands. The powder is also a particulate that could find its' way into your CSP. Therefore, pharmacy technicians use non-powdered gloves instead.

PROCEDURE

Removing Contaminated Gloves (Fig. 6-2)

1. To remove gloves, grasp the glove of your nondominant hand at the palm. Avoid grasping the glove at the wrist—you might transfer contaminants from your glove to your wrist. Make sure your hands are pointed down and away from your body.

2. Tug the glove toward the fingertips of your nondominant hand.

3. Slide your nondominant hand out of the glove by rolling against the palm of your dominant hand. You must be careful not to touch either glove with your bare hand.

4. Keep holding the soiled glove in the palm of your dominant hand. Slip your bare fingers under the cuff of the glove you're still wearing.

5. Stretch the glove of the dominant hand up and away from your hand. At the same time, turn the glove inside out. The glove you removed first should be balled up inside. The first glove should be inside the second glove, and the second glove should be inside out.

6. Discard the gloves as they are (without taking them apart) in a biohazard waste bin.

7. Wash your hands. Wearing gloves doesn't replace the need for proper hand washing!

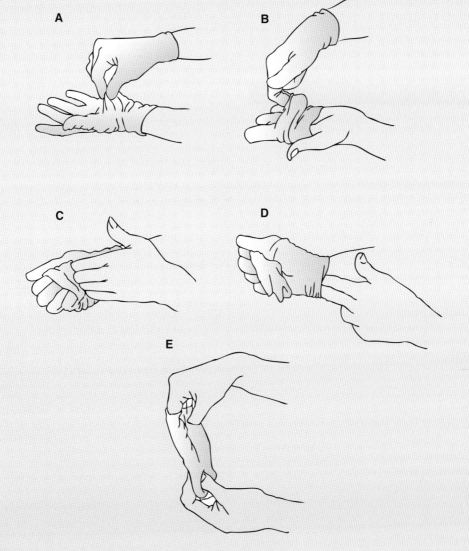

FIGURE 6-2 Grasp the palm of the glove on your non-dominant gloved hand (A). Carefully remove the glove and avoid contaminating your bare skin (B). Grasp the soiled glove with your gloved dominant hand (C). Slip your free hand under the cuff of the remaining glove (D). Remove the glove by turning it inside out over the previously removed glove (E).

CHAPTER HIGHLIGHTS

- The proper garbing order is scrubs (if necessary), shoe covers, head cover, beard cover, face mask, gown, gloves, and then eye shields. But, hand washing must be completed before gowns, gloves, and eye shields are put on.
- Wearing low-particulate garb when preparing CSPs helps keep the risk of contamination low.
- Careful hand washing removes nearly all bacteria commonly found on the hands.
- Antimicrobial agents include soaps such as Hibiclens, Vionex, and chlorohexidene gluconate.
- Proper hand-washing technique should take two to three minutes.
- Gloves may be sterile or non-sterile, powdered or non-powdered, latex or non-latex. Sterile, non-powdered gloves are used in the clean room area. Non-latex are used when sensitivity to latex.
- Follow the proper procedure for removing polluted gloves to avoid contaminating your skin.

QUICK QUIZ

Answer the following multiple-choice questions.

1. What does PPE stand for?
   a. protecting products in the environment
   b. personal product enrichment
   c. prioritizing personnel equipment
   d. personnel protective equipment
2. In which location will you find a pair of dedicated shoes?
   a. in the ante-area
   b. between the ante-area and clean room
   c. in the clean room
   d. inside an airflow hood
3. Which item should you dispose of immediately after leaving the clean room?
   a. dedicated shoes
   b. eye shield
   c. gown
   d. face mask
4. When do you put on your gown?
   a. before you wash your hands
   b. after you wash your hands
   c. before you put on shoe covers
   d. after you put on shoe covers
5. What type of glove should be used while compounding sterile products?
   a. sterile and powder-free
   b. latex and powder-free
   c. sterile and powdered
   d. powdered and latex-free

Please answer each of the following questions in one to three sentences.

1. Describe two items of PPE used by pharmacy technicians.
   _____
   _____

2. In what situations are non-latex gloves used?
   _____
   _____

3. Following the proper hand washing technique, what is the correct way to dry your hands?
   _____
   _____

4. What is an antimicrobial agent and when is it used?
   _____
   _____

5. What are three things to remember in regard to hand washing?
   _____
   _____

Label the following statements as either true or false.

1. ____ CSP compounding takes place in an area known as the ante-area.
2. ____ A gown must be discarded immediately after one-time use.
3. ____ The inside of powdered gloves are dusted with cornstarch.
4. ____ The entire hand washing process should take one to two minutes.
5. ____ Chlorohexidene gluconate is an alcohol-based cleaner used to disinfect gloves.

Match the term in the left column with the correct description from the right column.

1. chlorohexidene gluconate
2. PPE
3. cornstarch
4. antimicrobial soap
5. scrubs

a. the various pieces of clothing and gear worn by pharmacy technicians to lower the risk of personal infection and the spread of contamination
b. a specific product used to wash hands
c. short-sleeved garb item
d. an agent that kills microscopic pathogens
e. substance used inside powdered gloves

CHAPTER 7

Making Sterile Preparations

CHAPTER OBJECTIVES

- Identify and describe the different risk levels of CSPs.
- Evaluate the proper needle entry technique into a vial, ampule, and IV bag injection port.
- Determine how to use positive and negative pressure when compounding CSPs.
- Describe where, when, and what type of alcohol to use when compounding CSPs.
- Identify the correct sequence of steps in making a straight draw from a vial.
- Outline the process of reconstituting a powder.
- Explain how to remove bubbles from a syringe to draw accurate amounts of fluid.
- Determine how to package, label, and store CSPs.

KEY TERMS

closed-system containers—receptacles in which air cannot flow freely in or out

coring—transferring a part of the rubber stopper of a vial or container into a solution because of improper needle stick

endotoxins—compounds found inside infectious agents such as bacteria

media-fill test—an assessment that simulates the most challenging and stressful conditions under which you'll compound a CSP

negative pressure—a condition that occurs when the pressure outside a vial or bottle is greater than the pressure inside of it

open-system container—a receptacle in which air can pass freely in and out

positive pressure—a condition that occurs when the pressure inside a vial or bottle is greater than the pressure outside of it

risk level—the potential threat to patients caused by the introduction of microbial contamination into a finished sterile product

terminally sterilize—a process used to produce sterility in a final product contained in it's final packaging system

transfer needles—syringes that have needles on both ends

Viaflex bags— plastic, sterile IV containers that are not open to contaminants

There are many different ways to compound sterile preparations for use depending on the type of drug and size of order that you must fill. You'll prepare some of these medications using a syringe and filter needle or straw to withdraw from an ampule, and then, transfer to an IV bag. Others, you'll have to reconstitute from a powder to a liquid in a vial. Most often, you will package these in IV bags or syringes. Regardless of the process, you'll have to remember aseptic technique and be aware of risk levels—the underpinnings of sterile product preparation.

In this chapter, you'll learn to identify the risk levels assigned to sterile products regulated by the USP. You'll also learn a variety of procedures for manipulating needles, syringes, vials, and ampules and how to balance positive and negative pressure when preparing CSPs. Finally, you'll learn the proper procedures for labeling, storing, and transporting sterile products.

RISK LEVELS

One of the most important things to consider when preparing CSPs is the potential risk to patients if you contaminate a product. The USP provides clear and concise guidelines to determine the **risk level**—the potential threat to patients caused by the introduction of microbial contamination into a finished sterile product. It is the responsibility of the pharmacist to determine the risk level for each CSP. There are four specific categories:

- immediate-use
- low-risk
- low-risk with 12-hour or less BUD
- medium-risk
- high-risk

The USP assigned these risk levels based on the likelihood that a CSP will be contaminated by microbial contamination such as:

- spores
- **endotoxins**—compounds found inside infectious agents such as bacteria
- foreign chemicals (for example, cleaning supplies)
- physical matter (for example, lint, skin particles, hair, etc.)

When you know the risk level assigned to a product you're preparing, consider the source and quality of the ingredients you use, as well as the environmental and processing conditions.

Immediate-Use

The immediate-use risk level is a special designation. The USP designates this level for emergency situations in which a patient needs a product immediately, such as in:

- cardiopulmonary resuscitation
- emergency department treatment
- diagnostic agent preparation
- critical therapy, when there is additional risk involved in delaying treatment

All of the following criteria must be met to classify a CSP as immediate-use:

- Process must involve the simple transfer of not more than three commercially manufactured packages of sterile nonhazardous products
- Compounding procedure must be a continuous process that is completed in not more than one hour
- Aseptic technique is used
- Administration must begin within one hour of the start of the preparation process
- If not the person who prepared the CSP does not administer or witness the administration process, the CSP must be labeled
- If administration does not begin within one hour following the start of the preparation process, the CSP must be discarded

You shouldn't store or prepare immediate-use CSPs in batches in anticipation of future need. In fact, you should compound these products, from start to finish, within one hour. Although they're last-minute preparations, you should still maintain the highest level of sterility as possible.

Patient care-takers should administer an immediate-use CSP within one hour of the time you begin preparing it. Otherwise, you should discard it according to your facility's safe practice guidelines. Compounding in conditions that are higher than ISO class 5 increases the chance of microbial contamination. This could lead to patient harm, especially if the patient is critically ill or has a weak immune system.

Low-Risk

Low-risk CSPs have the lowest potential for contamination. You'll prepare these products in an ISO class 5 environment using aseptic preparation techniques. The initial ingredients are always sterile and in the manufacturer's original packaging.

Some examples of low-risk compounding include:

- single-volume transfers from ampules, bottles, bags, and vials using sterile syringes with sterile needles
- simple aseptic measuring and transferring with no more than three packages of manufactured sterile products (such as an infusion to compound drug admixtures)

You should store low-risk CSPs in a temperature-regulated setting. The guidelines indicate that you shouldn't store low-risk products longer than:

- 48 hours at controlled room temperature
- 14 days at a cold temperature
- 45 days in a solid frozen state

Low-Risk with 12-hour or Less BUD

It is not always feasible or practical to have CSPs prepared in a clean room. At times, CSPs must be prepared in a satellite pharmacy within a facility in order to get the medication to the patient more efficiently. When the PEC cannot be located in an ISO Class 7 buffer area, CSPs can still be prepared, but there are specific criteria that must be met. If the criteria are met, the CSP must be administered within 12 hours, or less if recommended by the manufacturer. If administration has not begun within 12 hours, then the preparation must be discarded.

All of the following criteria must be met in order to classify a CSP as Low-risk with 12-hour or less BUD:

- The PEC must be certified and maintain an ISO Class 5 environment, and located in a segregated compounding area specific for sterile product preparation

- The segregated compounding area cannot be located directly next to any unsealed windows or doors that would connect the area to the outdoors, the area must be low traffic, and the area must not be directly next to areas that would generate particles in the air (such as, a construction site, warehouse or cafeteria)
- The personnel preparing the CSPs must wash their hands and garb as though they were working in a clean room
- The segregated compounding area must be cleaned, disinfected and monitored just like a clean room, and the personnel must be trained and evaluated routinely like those working in a clean room

Medium-Risk

Although you prepare medium-risk CSPs in ISO Class 5 conditions, there will be several opportunities for contamination, for example, when:

- you prepare multiple small doses of CSPs that you combine to prepare a product that caretakers will administer to multiple patients or to one patient multiple times
- compounding involves complex aseptic manipulations other than single-volume transfers
- compounding requires an extended amount of time to complete

Some examples of medium-risk CSPs include:

- total parenteral nutrition fluids
- reservoirs of injection and infusion fluids
- volumes of a product that you transfer from multiple ampules or vials to a final sterile container

You'll store medium-risk CSPs in specific, regulated temperatures. The guidelines indicate that medium-risk products shouldn't be stored longer than:

- 30 hours in controlled room temperature
- 9 days in cold temperature
- 45 days in a frozen solid state

High-Risk

As a technician working to preserve the sterility and purity of compounded products, it's difficult to accept that contamination might occur.

However, with high-risk CSPs, it's a given that you're either starting with contaminated products or that you'll contaminate the products with which you're working. Some examples of high-risk sterile compounding include:

- dissolving nonsterile nutrient powders to make solutions that you'll **terminally sterilize**—a process

used to produce sterility in a final product contained in it's final packaging system
- exposing sterile ingredients to room air quality higher than ISO Class 5 for more than one hour
- measuring and mixing sterile ingredients in nonsterile devices
- storing nonsterile, water-containing preparations for more than six hours before sterilization

High-risk CSPs have rigid regulations in regard to storage. The guidelines indicate they shouldn't be stored longer than:

- 24 hours in controlled room temperature
- 3 days in cold temperature
- 45 days in a frozen solid state

Quality Control

Regardless of risk level, there are quality control measures that must be taken to ensure the purity and sterility of CPS.

Quality control should include:

- routinely disinfecting surfaces in the clean room
- visually confirming that all technicians are wearing the proper items and protective garments
- reviewing all orders and packages to ensure that orders and quantities are correct
- visually inspecting the CSPs to ensure that there is no particulate matter in solutions, no leakage from vials and bags, and labels are accurate and complete

In addition, **media-fill testing** should be performed by each personnel authorized to compound CSPs. The media-fill testing must be done annually for all risk levels except for high-risk, which must be performed semiannually. The media-fill test should simulate the most challenging or stressful conditions under which a person would prepare a CSP, therefore, high-risk media-fill tests are more challenging than low-risk media-fill test.

The topic of quality control or quality assurance is a very important one, and it will be covered in more detail in Chapter 9.

NEEDLE ENTRY

An obvious source of contamination during the preparation of sterile products is a syringe. As you learned in Chapter 4, you'll use needles in combination with a variety of containers:

- vials
- ampules
- IV bag injection ports

Since these storage units contain sterile products, disinfecting the needles with 70% sterile IPA before they

PROCEED WITH CAUTION

Avoid Coring

To avoid coring, insert the needle into the rubber stopper with the bevel tip up, and then apply slight lateral and downward pressure simultaneously to insert the needle (Fig. 7-1). You should start at a 30 degree angle with the bevel up. As you begin to insert the needle tip into the rubber, shift to a 90 degree angle and continue with downward pressure until the needle has completely punctured the rubber stopper. This should reduce the likelihood of contamination from rubber particles. This technique will take some practice.

contact the surface of the containers is a crucial step. In addition, there is a specific needle technique involved in extracting fluids from each of these units.

Extracting from Vials

The manufacturer maintains certain standards that ensure the sterility of the product in the vial. The point of transfer between the product in the vial and another receptacle, such as an IV bag, is the needle.

It is your responsibility to ensure the sterility of the rubber stopper on the top of the vial—the part of the vial that you'll puncture with a needle. You should carefully swab this area with 70% sterile IPA.

You learned in Chapter 4 that when you puncture a vial with a needle, you may contaminate the product with rubber. This is known as **coring**—transferring a

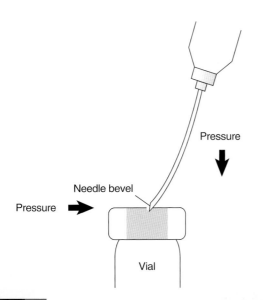

FIGURE 7-1 Proper needle insertion to prevent coring. (With permission from Thompson, J. E. (2009). *A Practical Guide to Contemporary Pharmacy Practice*. 3rd Ed. Baltimore, MD: Wolters Kluwer Health/Lippincott Williams & Wilkins.)

part of the rubber stopper of a vial or container into a solution because of improper needle stick

Extracting from Ampules

The process of removing fluid from an ampule is easy. Just tilt the ampule down slightly so that you can place the bevel tip of a needle on the inside bottom corner, or shoulder, of the ampule. Once the bevel tip is covered by the fluid, pull back on the syringe's plunger. This will draw the solution into the syringe.

There's always a chance, however, that the ampule will shed fine glass particles into the solution during the extracting process. In this case, you'll have to filter it. There are several different ways to do this:

- into a syringe through a filter needle, then switch to a regular needle and continue
- into a syringe through a regular needle, then switch to a filter needle and continue
- into a filter straw (used for tall ampoules or a large volume from one or more ampoules), then switch to a regular needle

It is very important that you filter when removing fluid from an ampule. It is easy to get confused if you do it differently each time you are withdrawing, therefore, it is best if you decide to always filter at the same time in your process. So, decide to always filter when withdrawing from the ampule or always filter after withdrawing from the ampule – just don't get yourself confused and forget to filter.

Extracting from IV Bag Injection Ports

Viaflex bags, are plastic, sterile IV containers that are not open to contaminants. The only penetrable opening on a viaflex bag is the injection port, which is at one end of the IV bag. The injection port allows for the addition of medications to a patient's IV solution. As always, the first step is to clean the injection port with a 70% sterile IPA wipe.

There are two layers of protection from contamination at the injection port site: the outside diaphragm and the inside diaphragm. When you're injecting a solution through the port into an IV bag (Fig. 7-2), make sure that the needle penetrates both the exterior and interior diaphragms. You will enter this port at a 90 degree angle. Be careful that you do not go in at an angle or the needle will exit the port. After depressing the plunger and removing the needle from the port, dispose the syringe properly in a sharps container.

PRESSURE IN A VIAL

All vials are **closed-system containers**—receptacles in which air cannot flow freely in or out. Any change in the

Negative Pressure

Removing too much air or fluid from a vial creates a vacuum. This is known as **negative pressure**—a condition that occurs when the pressure outside a vial or bottle is greater than the pressure inside of it. If too much negative pressure is present, it's difficult to remove the contents of the vial in an aseptic manner.

To keep the pressure as equal as possible, replace the volume of fluid removed from the vial with a slightly smaller volume of air to minimize the negative pressure.

It's always better to have a bit more negative pressure than positive pressure because it makes for a cleaner withdrawal of fluid.

T I P It's important when determining the pressure in a vial to remember that gas-producing drugs, such as chemotherapy drugs, will increase the positive pressure in a vial. You shouldn't add air to vials containing these medications after making a withdrawal.

MANIPULATION TECHNIQUE

The primary goal of learning proper manipulation technique is to keep CSPs, sterile instruments, equipment, and staff free of microbial contamination. As a pharmacy technician, you'll be performing procedures involving vials and ampules on a daily basis.

Alcohol

As you've already learned, 70% sterile IPA is one of the primary disinfectants in the clean room environment and is useful for disinfecting anything that will come into contact with the sterile product. Areas that you must wipe with alcohol include:

■ vial tops
■ ampule necks
■ tops of bottles
■ IV bag injection ports

Swabbing an area with alcohol works by:

■ removing physical contaminants
■ disinfecting as it evaporates—a process known as desiccation

Swabbing technique

Alcohol pads have many functions, but there's a proper way to apply them to guarantee sterility. First, place the alcohol pad on the area that you are cleaning, allowing the surface to become saturated. Then wipe gently once across the area. Allow the alcohol to dry completely before proceeding. You may reuse an alcohol pad if you have several ports or rubber stoppers to swab, but

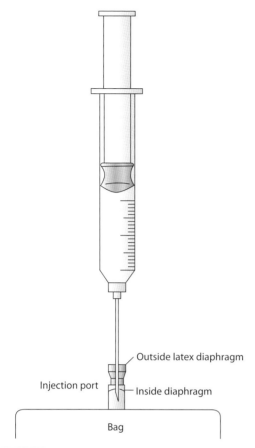

FIGURE 7-2 Technique for penetrating an IV injection port. (With permission from Thompson, J. E. (2009). *A Practical Guide to Contemporary Pharmacy Practice*. 3rd Ed. Baltimore, MD: Wolters Kluwer Health/Lippincott Williams & Wilkins.)

Labels: Outside latex diaphragm; Injection port; Inside diaphragm; Bag

amount of air or fluid within the vial will lead to positive or negative pressure within the vial.

Positive Pressure

Adding air or fluid to the vial will pressurize the vial, which is known as **positive pressure**—a condition that occurs when the pressure inside a vial or bottle is greater than the pressure outside of it. Positive pressure can cause:

■ spraying of the fluid from the vial
■ the vial to leak

You must equalize the pressure in a vial as much as possible after extracting fluid. Before withdrawing liquid from the vial, inject approximately the same amount of air into the vial as the amount of fluid that you will be extracting. This will stabilize the pressure. If the vial feels as though it is become over-pressurized and it is difficult to inject all of the air, inject some air and then let the vial equal by withdrawing some fluid before injecting more air. You can see-saw back and forth with the air and the fluid until you have removed the amount of fluid that you need.

PROCEDURE

Performing a Straight Draw

1. Wipe the rubber top of the vial with alcohol and allow it to dry (Fig. 7-3A).
2. Ensure that the needle is firmly attached to the syringe (Fig. 7-3B).
3. Pull the plunger back and forth to lubricate the barrel, then pull the plunger back on the syringe to slightly less than the amount of solution you need to draw (Fig 7-3C).
4. Remove the needle cap. Find the center of the stopper on top of the vial, and hold the needle with the bevel end facing up at a 30 degree angle (Fig. 7-3D).

5. As you begin to enter the rubber stopper, swing the needle up to a 90 degree angle and fully enter the vial (Fig 7-3E).
6. Invert the vial and needle without shadowing, and slowly push the air from the syringe into the vial (Fig. 7-3F).
7. Pull back on the plunger until you withdraw the desired amount from the vial (Fig 7-3G).
8. Remove any air bubbles from the syringe. (You'll learn more about this later in the chapter.)
9. Invert the vial and needle without shadowing, withdraw the needle and carefully recap the end, or inject it into the IV bag injection port and slowly inject.

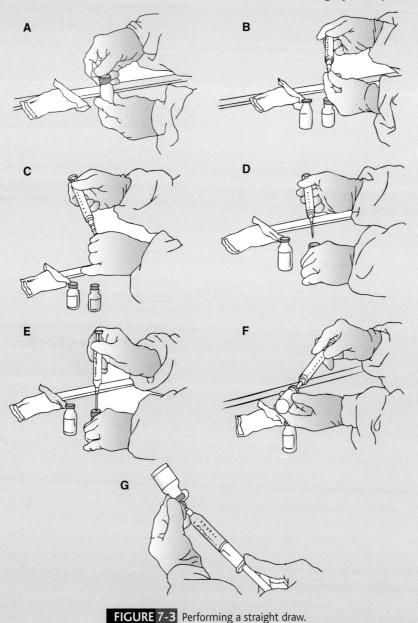

FIGURE 7-3 Performing a straight draw.

it is important to use a different corner or surface for each one.

Vial Manipulation

Vials are useful for sterile storage of medications, both liquid and powder, and you'll use them regularly when preparing CSPs. Considering that vials are closed systems, there are specific guidelines in place to help you accurately and safely:

- perform a straight draw
- reconstitute a powder
- remove air bubbles
- use a transfer needle

Straight Draw Technique

Performing a straight draw of solution from a vial is one of the simplest and most common manipulations you'll be required to do. With a few substitutions in procedure, you can use it in nearly all manipulations when preparing CSPs.

Remember that you must do a straight draw procedure in a clean air space (such as the laminar airflow hood) using the proper aseptic technique.

Now that you know how to perform a straight draw, you'll be able to conduct many necessary manipulations when preparing CSPs. Let's take a look at how to prepare a powdered product in a vial.

Reconstituting a Powder

Sometimes you'll find that a manufacturer will only supply a drug in a vial in powdered form. In order to transfer and use these drugs, you must first reconstitute them.

PROCEDURE

Reconstituting a Powder

1. Wipe the rubber top of the vials with alcohol and let them dry.
2. Make sure the needle is firmly attached to the syringe.
3. Insert the needle into the vial of the diluent (same as a straight draw), and withdraw the correct amount of diluent that you need to reconstitute the powder.
4. Pull back the plunger to clear the neck of the syringe. This empties all of the fluid from the needle into the syringe.
5. Remove the needle and replace it with a vented needle.
6. Insert the vented needle into the vial of the powder (as a straight draw) making sure that the vent on the needle is inside the vial. Slowly add the diluent to the powder in the vial. (If you do not have a vented

needle, you can use a regular needle; however, you must remove an equal volume of air to prevent the positive pressure from building up.)
7. Gently shake or swirl the vial to dissolve the powder completely.
8. Reswab the rubber stopper if you feel that you shadowed or might have otherwise contaminated it during the reconstitution process.
9. Obtain a new syringe or exchange the vented needle with a regular needle, and carefully withdraw the desired amount of reconstituted drug from the vial.
10. Remove any air bubbles from the syringe. (You'll learn more about this later in the chapter.)
11. Recap the needle, or insert the needle into the IV bag injection port, and slowly inject.

Remember, to reconstitute a powder you add a diluent to the vial to create a liquid. The diluent is usually sterile water for injection, but the vial's packaging instructions will indicate exactly what to use. The following Procedure describes how to reconstitute a powder.

TIP Although swirling the vial will usually dissolve all of the powder, you need to make sure that the drug is completely suspended before you continue. To do this, simply inspect the contents visually to make sure there are no particles or clumps. You must also make sure there are no coring fragments that might have broken off when you punctured the rubber top of the vial. If you find any particulate matter in the solution, you'll need to filter the solution before proceeding.

Removing Air Bubbles

One of the most important methods to ensure that you have drawn the accurate amount of fluid is to eliminate any air bubbles that may be in the syringe. When you're working with extremely small amounts, such as a fraction of a milliliter, any air in the syringe can greatly affect the amount of drug you draw.

There's a simple technique for removing air bubbles from a syringe. It's a good idea to make these simple steps a habit each time you draw a solution into a syringe.

Transfer Needles

Transfer needles are syringes that have needles on both ends. These are especially useful when transferring the entire contents of a vial into an IV bag. The following Procedure describes how to use transfer needles.

Ampule Manipulation

Ampules are different from vials in that they're made entirely of glass. Once you open an ampule, it becomes

Removing Air Bubbles

1. Draw back on the plunger to allow more fluid into the syringe.
2. Carefully rotate the large air bubble around the syringe to pick-up the smaller air bubbles.
3. If any air bubbles remain, carefully tap the syringe with your knuckles to dislodge the smaller air bubbles.
4. Hold the syringe upright and pull the plunger back another 0.2 mL to clear the hub.
5. Carefully push the plunger up to remove the air. Make sure all air has been removed from the needle because depending on the size of the needle it can hold up to 0.1 mL of air.
6. Check to make sure that the desired amount of drug is in the syringe.
7. If you need to adjust the volume, you may do so bevel down onto an alcohol swab or sterile gauze pad making sure to not shadow or spray into the HEPA filter.

Using Transfer Needles

1. Wipe the appropriate areas (IV injection port and rubber top of the vial) with an alcohol swab.
2. Place the longer of the two needles into the IV bag injection port.
3. Place the shorter of the two needles into the vial.
4. Gently squeeze the IV bag, causing the IV fluid to slowly fill the vial.
5. Shake the vial gently so that the powder dissolves completely.
6. Hold the IV bag so that all of the air floats to the top. Then gently squeeze the bag so the air will move into the vial, creating positive pressure. The pressure will force the fluid down into the IV bag.
7. Make sure that you have forced all the fluid from the vial into the bag before removing the transfer syringe.
8. Remove the transfer needle from the IV bag injection port first, maintaining the closed system.
9. Remove the transfer needle from the vial and dispose it properly in a sharps container.

an **open-system container**—a receptacle in which air can pass freely in and out. You can only use an ampule once, unlike multi-dose vials, which you can use many times.

Removing Air Bubbles

Before you open an ampule, you should make sure that all of the fluid moves from the head of the ampule (the top part) to the body (the lower part). You can do this by:

- swirling the ampule in an upright motion
- tapping the head of the ampule with a finger
- inverting the ampule and quickly swinging it back into an upright position

Breaking the Ampule Neck

You should only break open an ampule toward the side of the hood. If you break it toward the back of the hood,

glass particles could enter the HEPA filter, which can cause damage to the filter. If you have trouble opening the ampule, try rotating it a half-turn so that the pressure on the neck is at a different angle.

TIP When you're preparing to open an ampule, first swab the neck with 70% sterile IPA and allow the alcohol to dry. You may then either use a clean alcohol swab to help you open the ampule, or use your hand. Placing a clean alcohol swab on the neck of the ampule. has a two-fold use. First, it helps prevent you from cutting your finger when you break the neck, and second, it minimizes the amount of glass particles and drug that may spray upon opening. However, the alcohol also make the gloves and the ampule somewhat slippery and makes it more difficult to open for some. Try both techniques and see which one works best for you.

 PROCEED WITH CAUTION

Closed System Only

When you're removing air bubbles from a syringe, you must make sure that the environment is a closed system to ensure than no contaminants enter the solution through the needle. If you're drawing the solution from a vial, leave the needle in the vial while eliminating the air bubbles if possible.

 PROCEED WITH CAUTION

One-Time-Use Needles

You can only use filter needles once, so always switch the filter needle with a regular needle once you've drawn the fluid into the syringe. Otherwise, you may inject the filtered objects into the IV bag, which would negate the filtering effect and contaminate the solution in the bag.

Withdrawing Fluid from an Ampule

1. Remove the air bubbles from the body of the ampule.
2. Swab the neck of the ampule and the IV injection port of the bag with 70% sterile IPA and allow the alcohol to dry.
3. Hold the ampule at a 20° angle toward the side of the hood.
4. Apply pressure with your thumbs toward the neck of the ampule using a hands away motion. It is important to move the hands apart when opening the ampule to avoid bringing the thumb holding the top of the ampule back across the body of the ampule which might have a glass shard sticking up.
5. Attach a filter needle or straw to the syringe.
6. Withdraw the fluid from the ampule. You can hold the ampule parallel to the work surface or slightly inverted. The surface tension, in most cases, will prevent the fluid from spilling out of the ampule.
7. Empty the needle or straw into the syringe clearning the hub of the syringe. Change the needle or straw to a regular needle
8. Remove any air bubbles and adjust to the correct volume.
9. Insert the needle into the IV injection port and slowly inject the fluid.

Withdrawing Fluid from an Ampule

As with all other manipulations, you should only withdraw fluid from an ampule in an ISO Class 5 PEC using proper aseptic techniques. Use the following steps to ensure a successful withdraw.

Injecting into IV Bottles

Injecting into an IV bottle is slightly different than injecting into a bag. You will still need to clean the rubber stopper with 70% sterile IPA before injecting. However, when you insert the needle into the bottle, you will find that the bottle is vacuum packed and will pull the fluid from the syringe into the bottle with little effort on your part. Make sure all of the fluid has been injected from the syringe into the bottle and remove the needle and discard.

PACKAGING

Drug manufacturers include package inserts and instructions with the products that they prepare. The packaging provides storage, usage, BUD, and preparation information necessary to properly use the product.

Once you create new CSPs, you should label the products and seal them properly. You must also take into account whether or not the product is a chemotoxic or hazardous material.

Labeling

Accurate labels assure that everyone knows a product's components and instructions for use. The USP and ASHP provide clear instructions for how you should properly label a CSP. Sterile products must include the following information:

- the patient's name or other patient ID (for patient-specific products)
- control or lot numbers
- all solution and ingredient names, amounts, strengths, and concentrations
- the total volume
- the prescribed administration regimen
- expiration date
- time of preparation (if it's an immediate-use drug)
- auxiliary labeling
- storage requirements (temperature, light-sensitivity, etc.)
- identification of the responsible pharmacist
- device-specific instructions

You might have to include additional information, such as reference numbers, depending on state and federal regulations.

Tamper-Evident Closures and Seals

Maintaining the integrity of the prepared CSP is of utmost importance, especially once it leaves the compounding facility. One way to ensure that there has been no breach of the sterile container is through the use of tamper-evident closures and seals on CSP ports. These provide an extra measure of security regardless of how staff transports or handles the products. When patient care takers receive a sealed CSP, they're more confident in your work and in administering the drug to their patients.

Chemotoxic and Hazardous Drugs

Because of their sensitive nature, chemotoxic and other hazardous CSPs require additional safeguards to ensure their stability. It's your job to minimize their potential exposure to the environment and to those who come into contact with them.

Special requirements associated with the packaging, transporting, and handling of these CSPs include preventing accidental spills or exposure. You can do this by:

- using Luer-lock syringes and connections
- using syringe caps
- capping container ports
- using sealed plastic bags
- implementing impact-resistant containers
- using cautionary labeling

TRANSPORTING

So far, you have learned many ways to assure the sterility and accuracy of the products you'll be compounding. It is also important to take additional measures to guarantee their safety while they're transported. These measures take into account several factors:

- protection in packaging
- reliable transit
- CSPs of special circumstance

Protection in Packaging

When you're shipping CSPs outside of the compounding facility, you must select packing containers that will maintain the physical integrity, sterility, and stability of the CSPs during transit. The packing you select should protect the products from:

- damage
- leaks
- contamination
- degradation

Each compounding facility has standard operating procedures that will outline specifically the appropriate packing containers and stuffing materials. You'll acquire this information from:

- product specifications
- vendors
- past experience of compounding technicians

You should always check to make sure that the recipients receive written instructions on how to safely open containers of packed CSPs.

Transportation Conditions

It's the job of the compounding facility to select and review competent and reliable transportation services for the transport of CSPs. Services should assure your facility that the packages will arrive undamaged, still in their sterile and stable condition.

Temperature is the most important component of safe transporting. The temperature during transit cannot exceed the warmest temperature specified on the storage temperature range on CSP labels. The compounding facility should contact the courier to ensure appropriate conditions are possible.

Special Circumstances

Some circumstances involve products that require special handling or transport. Some of these are:

- pneumatic tube systems
- chemotoxic and hazardous drugs

Pneumatic Tube Systems

You should encase CSPs that are administered through pneumatic tube systems in foam padding or inserts to make sure they don't break. Shaking that occurs during transportation could affect the stability of the preparation. Therefore, evaluate each product on a case-by-case basis.

Chemotoxic and Hazardous Drugs

Chemotoxic and hazardous drugs require even more delicate handling. Avoid transporting these CSPs by pneumatic tubing because of the potential for breakage and contamination. These types of drugs require special arrangements and preparation to handle events such as spills and exposure.

REDISPENSING STERILE PRODUCTS

You must evaluate CSPs that pharmacies or hospitals return to the compounding facility to determine whether they're able to be dispensed again. Of course, these CSPs must not be open or display evidence of tampering, and you must be able to ensure that the products:

- were maintained at the correct temperature
- are returned within the timeframe of the original BUD

ASSESSING ASEPTIC TECHNIQUE, SAFETY, AND QUALITY ASSURANCE PRACTICES

The USP Chapter 797 provides a checklist (see next page) to help you follow aseptic technique, safety, and quality assurance practices. The checklist is both an evaluation tool for your superiors and a guide to self-check as you're learning to follow all of the steps involved in preparing sterile products.

Eventually, through practice and experience, these self-checks will become second nature to you. Here's the checklist:

Not all of the criteria on the checklist will be applicable with every compounding assignment, but it's good practice to be familiar with all of the safeguard requirements.

CHAPTER HIGHLIGHTS

- The USP has designed four specific categories of risk levels for sterile compounding: immediate-use, low- (including low-risk with 12-hour or less BUD), medium-, and high-risk.
- There are variations in the storage requirements and quality control of each risk level.
- Making straight draws from vials is a common and simple procedure.

Checklist for Assessing the Aseptic Technique, Safety, and Quality Assurance of Compounding Personnel

MARK EACH SPACE BELOW WITH A CHECK IF SATISFACTORILY COMPLETED

_____ Performs hand hygiene and garbing procedures according to standard operating procedures

_____ Disinfects ISO Class 5 device surfaces with an appropriate agent

_____ Disinfects components/vials with an appropriate agent before placing in an ISO Class 5 work area

_____ Introduces only essential materials in a proper arrangement in the ISO Class 5 work area

_____ Does not interrupt, impede, or divert the flow of first air to critical sites

_____ Ensures that syringes, needles, and tubing remain in their individual packaging and are only opened in an ISO Class 5 work area

_____ Performs manipulations only in the direct compounding area of the ISO Class 5 device

_____ Does not expose critical sites to contact contamination or worse than ISO Class 5 air

_____ Disinfects stoppers, injection ports, and ampule necks by wiping with 70% sterile IPA and allows sufficient time to dry

_____ Affixes needles to syringes without contact contamination

_____ Punctures vial stoppers and penetrates injection ports without contact contamination

_____ Labels preparations correctly and completely

_____ Disinfects sterile gloves routinely by wiping with 70% sterile IPA during prolonged compounding manipulations

_____ Cleans, sets up, and calibrates automated compounding devices according to the manufacturer's instructions

_____ Disposes of sharps and waste according to institutional policy or recognized guidelines

---

- Eliminating pressure fluctuation within a vial can be done by adding or reducing the amount of air or liquid in the vial.
- All critical sites can be disinfected with 70% sterile IPA.
- Reconstituting a powder within a vial requires a few simple steps and careful measurements.
- Using ampules in compounding requires careful manipulation and a filter syringe.
- Proper labeling of a prepared CSP ensures that the product is stored and administered correctly.
- The staff of the compounding facility is responsible for ensuring the sterility, stability, and purity of all compounded products even after they've left the facility.
- The facility should take into account light sensitivity, temperature factors, and special-case CSPs when arranging transportation of products.

QUICK QUIZ

Answer the following multiple-choice questions.

1. You use a media-fill test to
   a. check the accuracy of the ingredients in a product.
   b. measure the amount of fluid in a vial or ampule.
   c. test the technique of compounding personnel
   d. test the amount of microbes in the air and surfaces of a clean room.

2. What must you do to all vials before withdrawing fluid from them?
   a. verify the expiration date
   b. swirl them to dissolve the contents
   c. bring them to room temperature
   d. swab the rubber tops with alcohol wipes

3. You would most likely use an immediate-use CSP during
   a. chemotherapy treatments.
   b. total parenteral nutrition administration.
   c. cardiopulmonary resuscitation.
   d. high-dose antibiotic treatments.

4. The solution you'll most commonly use for reconstitution is
   a. 5% dextrose.
   b. sodium chloride.
   c. normal saline.
   d. sterile water for injection.

5. Chemotoxic and other hazardous drugs shouldn't be transported by pneumatic tubing because
   a. they require refrigeration.
   b. they may break, causing dangerous contamination.
   c. they may not be delivered to the correct patient.
   d. they're immediate-use products.

Please answer each of the following questions in one to three sentences.

1. What are the three ways to remove air bubbles from an ampule before you open it?

_____

_____

2. Explain the difference between positive and negative pressure in a vial.

_____

_____

3. Why is it crucial to remove air bubbles from a syringe?

_____

_____

4. List the steps in performing a straight draw from a vial.

_____

_____

5. Name five things that you should include on the label of a CSP.

_____

_____

Label the following statements as either true or false.

1. ____ Once you open an ampule, it becomes an open system.
2. ____ You use Viaflex bags to transfer the contents of one syringe to another.
3. ____ Filter needles are one-time-use needles that you'll use when withdrawing solution from ampules.

4. ____ Negative pressure is a condition that occurs when the pressure inside a vial or bottle is greater than the pressure outside of it.
5. ____ Low-risk CSPs should have a lower potential for contamination compared to high-risk CSPs.

Match the term in the left column with the correct description from the right column.

1. endotoxins	a. the potential threat to patients caused by the introduction of microbial contamination into a finished sterile product
2. negative pressure	b. a condition that occurs when the pressure inside a vial or bottle is greater than the pressure outside of it
3. risk level	c. compounds found inside infectious agents such as bacteria
4. Viaflex bags	d. a condition that occurs when the pressure outside a vial or bottle is greater than the pressure inside of it
5. positive pressure	e. plastic, sterile IV containers that are not open to contaminants

CHAPTER 8

Basic Sterile Preparations

CHAPTER OBJECTIVES

- Identify the different types of CSPs.
- Define a hazardous drug.
- Identify the equipment that is needed to compound a hazardous drug CSP.
- Describe the environmental requirements for compounding a hazardous drug CSP.
- Explain the manipulation techniques for compounding a hazardous drug CSP in a BSC or CAI.
- Describe the environmental requirements and standards involved in compounding radiopharmaceuticals as CSPs.
- Explain the need for total parenteral nutrition (TPN).
- Identify fluids and electrolytes commonly used to compound a TPN.
- List the types, use and maintenance of automated compounding devices (ACD).

KEY TERMS

allergen extract—a biologic that is used to test for an allergy

antineoplastic—a chemical that slows down or prevents the growth and reproduction of cancerous cells

biologic—a substance produced by a living source

buffer—substance added to a solution or suspension to obtain a desired pH

chemo mat—a special device placed outside the BSC to absorb any leaks or spills

chemotherapy—the use of chemicals to treat a disease, especially cancer

closed system transfer device (CSTD)—a special system for transferring hazardous drugs from one container to another

cold chain—the steps taken to keep a biologic at a specific low temperature from the manufacturer's refrigerator to the pharmacy, clinic, or doctor's office where it is administered'

compounding aseptic containment isolator (CACI)—a CAI that is designed to protect the worker as well as the product; used to compound hazardous drugs

cytotoxic—a chemical that poisons cells so that they are not able to reproduce or grow

diabetes mellitus—disease which results when a person's body (specifically, the pancreas) does not produce enough insulin

dilution—a process that makes a more concentrated substance less concentrated

essential amino acids—amino acids which are not produced by the body and must therefore be supplied through the diet

hazardous drug—a drug that can cause serious effects such as cancer, organ toxicity, fertility problems, genetic damage, or birth defects

hemodialysis—type of dialysis used to remove toxic substances from the blood

insulin pump—lightweight pump that maintains blood glucose levels at a normal level

malignant—cancerous

peritoneal dialysis—type of dialysis in which a solution is allowed to flow into the peritoneal, or abdominal, cavity in order to remove toxic substances

PhaSeal—a type of CSTD that keeps human exposure to chemotherapy drugs to a minimum

precipitate—a solid mass that forms in a solution when two or more substances react

radiopharmaceutical—a radioactive CSP used in nuclear medicine to diagnose and treat certain diseases

rhinitis—the irritation and inflammation of the internal areas of the nose

technetium-99m (Tc-99m)—isotope commonly used for compounding radiopharmaceuticals

vaccination—the use of a biologic product, a vaccine, to produce active immunity in a patient

viscosity—how the fluid is able to flow

You have already learned many things about CSPs. You have learned how to prepare CSPs, how to prevent contamination, how to make calculations related to CSPs, what equipment is used to prepare CSPs, what a clean room is, what proper aseptic technique is, and how many sterile products are made.

In this chapter you will learn about different types of sterile preparations—biologics, hazardous drugs, radiopharmaceuticals, insulin, chemotherapy agents, insulin, injectable pellets, irrigations, nasal preparations, epidurals, ophthalmics, otic preparations, pediatric preparations, patient-controlled analgesics, proteins, and total parenteral nutrition products. You'll learn what these preparations are used for, how they are used, and other details that you will need to know as a pharmacy technician.

STERILE PREPARATIONS

There are many different kinds of compounded sterile preparations, or CSPs. How do you determine what a CSP is? According to USP chapter 797, all CSPs satisfy one of the following two conditions. A CSP is a dosage unit that is prepared according to manufacturer's directions, or is prepared from non-sterile ingredients that must be sterilized before administration.

Below is a list of the CSPs that will be described in this chapter:

- biologics
- chemotherapy agents
- dialysis products
- epidurals
- hazardous drugs and radiopharmaceuticals
- injectable pellets or implants
- insulin
- irrigations
- nasal preparations
- ophthalmics
- otic preparations
- pediatric preparations
- patient-controlled analgesics
- proteins
- total parenteral nutrition products

BIOLOGICS

A **biologic** is a CSP produced by a living source. A biologic product can be any virus, therapeutic serum toxin, antitoxin, or similar product used to prevent, treat, or cure a human disease. For example, many vitamins, hormones, and antibiotics are biologics.

USP chapter 797 discusses the role of the pharmacist and pharmacy technician with regard to CSPs. Generally, pharmacists and pharmacy technicians have the responsibility to prepare sterile preparations. USP 797 also points out that the highest standards of sterility are expected to be maintained when doing so.

Immunizations

You've probably had personal experience with immunizations, or vaccines. An immunization, or **vaccination**, is a biologic product (a vaccine) used to produce active immunity in a patient.

Pharmacists are able to work with physicians and nurses to immunize patients. As of the date of this publication, pharmacists in 37 states were able to give vaccinations. These include vaccines for influenza, diphtheria, tetanus, pertussis, measles, mumps, rubella, and polio.

Storage and Handling

A key role of the pharmacist is to properly train pharmacy technicians in the proper storage, handling, and shipping of biologic products so that the cold chain is maintained. The **cold chain** describes the steps taken to keep a biologic at a specific temperature. The cold chain must be maintained from the manufacturer's refrigerator to the pharmacy, clinic, or doctor's office. Most biologics are stored in a separate refrigerator at a temperature of 2-8 degrees Celsius. It is important that any biologic be maintained at a specific cold temperature in order for the product to remain effective. Therefore, the importance of following the steps of the cold chain is a critical task of the pharmacist and pharmacy technician.

Allergen Extracts

Another kind of biologic is an allergen extract. **Allergen extracts** are used to test for allergies. Allergen extracts, as CSPs, can be administered as a single dose or in multiple doses. They are usually given as either an intradermal or a subcutaneous injection.

Allergen extracts are not bound by the same storage requirements that are necessary for most CSP biologics. However, this is the case only if all of the following conditions are met:

- The allergen extract is compounded using a simple transfer with a sterile needle and syringe and commercial sterile allergen product.
- The allergen extract contains substances that prevent the growth of microorganisms.
- Before compounding allergen extracts, thorough hand-cleansing is performed for at least 30 seconds with an antimicrobial soap and water.
- Hair covers, facial hair covers, gowns, and/or face masks are worn.
- Antiseptic hand cleansing is performed using an alcohol-based surgical hand scrub.

- Powder-free sterile gloves are worn and wiped with 70% sterile IPA before beginning, and intermittently throughout compounding.
- Each multiple-dose vial of allergen extract lists the name of a specific patient as well as a beyond-use-date (BUD.)
- Ampule necks and vial stoppers are disinfected with 70% sterile IPA.
- Aseptic technique minimizes direct contact contamination.
- Single-dose allergen extracts are not stored for additional use.

HAZARDOUS DRUGS AND RADIOPHARMACEUTICALS

A special group of CSPs requires extreme caution and special handling. This group contains CSPs known as hazardous drugs. A **hazardous drug** is a drug that can cause serious negative effects such as cancer, organ toxicity, fertility problems, genetic damage, or birth defects. Hazardous drugs include:

- chemotherapy agents such as antineoplastics and cytotoxics
- radiopharmaceuticals
- immunosuppressive agents

To prevent exposure, hazardous drugs are prepared, administered, and disposed of in, at least an ISO Class 5 environment. The following equipment is used:

- closed system transfer devices
- a biological safety cabinet (BSC) or compounding aseptic isolator (CAI) that maintains an ISO Class 5 environment (no more than 100 particles per cubic foot) that is located in an ISO Class 7 (no more than 10,000 particles per cubic foot) buffer area within a negative pressure room
- chemotherapy gloves

Manipulation and Handling Techniques

The safest method for manipulating hazardous drugs is to use a **closed system transfer device (CSTD)**. This is a special system used for transferring hazardous drugs from one container to another. Transferring a particular amount of a hazardous drug from a vial to a syringe is an example. A CSTD prevents any venting or exposure of the hazardous drug to the environment.

It is also important that hazardous drugs be stored separately from other CSPs and drugs to prevent contamination in the event of a breakage or spillage. By following these specific guidelines, you, as the pharmacy technician, help protect yourself as well as other personnel in the preparation and storage areas.

Radiopharmaceuticals

One group of hazardous CSPs is the **radiopharmaceuticals**. These are radioactive CSPs used in nuclear medicine to diagnose and treat certain diseases. Many radiopharmaceuticals are compounded using the isotope **technetium-99m** (Tc-99m). Another commonly used radiopharmaceutical is strontium-89 chloride (Sr-89). The use of radiopharmaceuticals in nuclear imaging makes it possible to diagnose tumors and abnormalities of the brain, lungs and other body parts.

Special Handling

Special standards apply to the compounding of radiopharmaceuticals. These include:

- using shielded vials and/or syringes such as those in a CSTD
- working in a certified ISO Class 5 environment (no more than 100 particles per cubic foot) located in an ISO Class 8 (no more than 100,000 particles per cubic foot) air environment

Chemotherapy Agents

Cancer is a difficult disease that grows at different rates, behaves differently, and responds to different treatments. Unfortunately, there is no one treatment for cancer. Some cancers are treated by removing the cancerous, or **malignant**, cells. Others are treated with a type of hazardous drug known as a chemotherapy drug. The term **chemotherapy** refers to using chemicals to treat a disease. Generally, chemotherapy refers to treatment for cancer. However, chemotherapy is also used to treat rheumatoid arthritis, lupus, psoriasis, and other autoimmune diseases. Chemotherapy medications may be prepared in a syringe, an IVPB, or as a continuous infusion.

The chemicals used in chemotherapy treatments are described as cytotoxic or antineoplastic. **Cytotoxic** agents are chemicals that poison cells so that they are not able to reproduce or grow. **Antineoplastics** slow down or prevent the growth and reproduction of cancerous cells.

Special Equipment

The compounding of chemotherapy agents begins with a physician's order. Once the pharmacy receives the order, the pharmacist makes sure the order is written correctly. Then, the pharmacy technician prepares to compound the product.

Chemotherapy agents are prepared in a Class II BSC, also known as a vertical airflow hood, or a **compounding aseptic containment isolator (CACI)**. As you have already learned, this means that the airflow hood contains high-efficiency HEPA filters. The class II BSC protects you, the product, and the environment from the hazards associated with chemotherapy agents. It also prevents cross-contamination along the work surface of the BSC.

Additional equipment for compounding chemotherapy agents may include:

- biohazard waste containers
- spill kits
- special gloves
- shower apparatus
- dispensing pins

Another special device called a **chemo mat** can be placed inside the BSC to absorb any leaks or spills.

PhaSeal

When compounding hazardous drugs, you may use a CSTD called the **PhaSeal**. This is a closed system transfer device that keeps human exposure to chemotherapy drugs to a minimum. The PhaSeal is a set of disposable containment devices used in chemotherapy preparation. The PhaSeal connects the original drug vial, the syringe, and IV injection together in a sealed pathway.

Manipulation Techniques

The ASHP Technical Assistance Bulletin on Handling Cytotoxic and Hazardous Drugs lists valuable information about the safe handling of chemotherapy medications. Some of these tips include the following:

- Identify and label all chemotherapy drugs.
- Have a written procedure on-hand, as well as a chemo spill kit, for any chemo spills.
- Place chemo drugs in a bin, not on a shelf.
- Transport chemotherapy drugs using a cart with a rim.
- Maintain written policies and procedures for preparing all chemotherapy agents.
- Keep MSDS (Material Safety Data Sheets) for each chemotherapy drug within easy access.
- Make sure airflow and venting protects the sterility of the chemotherapy agent as well as personnel from possible exposure.
- Wear appropriate apparel including gloves (double gloving), gown, respirator, goggles.
- Always use proper aseptic technique.

Administration/Handling of Chemotherapy Agents

When handling cytotoxic agents, you should always follow aseptic technique. By carefully following the same step-by-step process, you help protect yourself and the product from contamination.

PROCEDURE

Withdrawing a Cytotoxic Agent Using a Regular Needle

1. Gather all materials needed.
2. Remember that the airflow in the BSC is downward. Never block the airflow—Do not place your hands or fingers between sterile items and the direction of airflow.
3. Swab the rubber top with 70% sterile IPA and allow it to dry.
4. Make sure the needle is firmly attached to the syringe.
5. Pull the syringe plunger back and forth to lubricate the barrel, then pull the plunger back to about half the amount of drug needed.
6. Remove the cap from the needle. Insert the needle in the center of the stopper, bevel end up.
7. Turn the vial on its side so that clean air can blow directly on the sterile parts of the syringe and stopper.
8. Hold the syringe on the bottom side. Slowly add the air from the syringe into the vial.
9. Remove the desired amount of cytotoxic agent by pulling back on the plunger.
10. Remove the needle from the vial when the desired amount of drug is withdrawn.
11. Remove any air bubbles using an empty container.
12. Recap the syringe.
13. Perform a final check.

Chemo Spills

There are two kinds of chemo spills—large and small. A small spill is defined as being less than 5 mL or 5 g. A large spill is anything over 5 mL or 5 g. A chemo spill kit should be located close to the preparation area. A spill is never planned, so having a chemo spill kit nearby, and knowing how to use it, is critically important.

These are the necessary items for your chemo spill kit:

- chemical splash goggles
- low-permeability disposable gown and shoe covers or coveralls
- two pairs of gloves (utility and latex)
- two sheets of absorbent, plastic-backed material
- 250-mL and 1-L spill control pillows
- puncture-resistant sharps container
- smalls coop to collect glass fragments
- two large, labeled, sealable hazardous drug waste disposal bags
- appropriate respirator

Disposal

Be sure to dispose of all chemotherapy agents and related items in a special yellow, puncture-resistant hazardous container (Fig. 8-1). The container should be labeled *Chemotherapy Waste Container*. Before placing items into this container, they should be sealed in a zip-lock bag. Needles and syringes should be placed, without clipping or capping them, in a standard puncture-proof sharps container. The kinds of items that are disposed of in this container include:

- gloves
- disposable gowns
- disposable goggles
- other disposable material used during chemotherapy administration (IV bags/bottles, tubing, and any unbreakable items)

DIALYSIS

Dialysis is a process that separates substances that are in solution. The separation is possible based on differences in the way the substances move through a membrane.

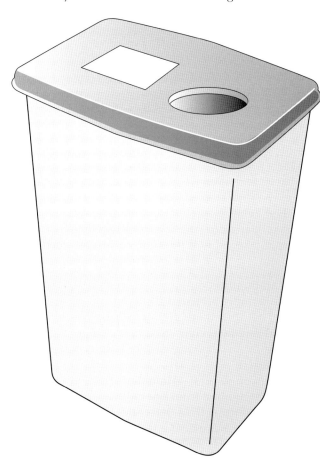

FIGURE 8-1 Throw all gloves, gown, goggles, and other disposable material used during chemotherapy administration into a designated, yellow, chemotherapy waste container.

(i.e., Some substances move through a membrane more easily than others.) Dialysis solutions are generally used in large volumes, so they come in large containers, like large IV bags.

There are two types of dialysis—peritoneal dialysis and hemodialysis. In **peritoneal dialysis**, a dialysis solution is allowed to flow into the peritoneal, or abdominal, cavity. A thin peritoneal membrane surrounds and protects the organs of the abdomen. This membrane acts as a blood filter by removing toxic substances from the blood and passing them into the dialysis solution. As the solution becomes filled with waste and toxins, it is exchanged for fresh dialysis fluid.

The other type of dialysis, **hemodialysis**, is used to remove toxic substances from the blood. Here's how hemodialysis works:

1. The blood is directed out of the body through an artery.
2. The blood passes through a polyethylene catheter.
3. The blood is cleaned of toxins and waste by passing it through a special artificial dialysis filter.
4. The blood is returned to the body through a vein.

IRRIGATIONS

Irrigation solutions are used to bathe or wash wounds, incisions, or body tissues. Like dialysis solutions, irrigations are not injected directly into a vein or artery. Instead, they are used outside the circulatory system.

Solutions

There are several types of irrigation solutions. A few commonly used irrigations solutions are:

- acetic acid irrigation, USP—used for irrigating the bladder, or for washing away blood or surgical debris.
- Ringer's Irrigation, USP—used to irrigate body surfaces, must be labeled NOT FOR INJECTION.
- sodium chloride irrigation, USP—used to wash wounds and body cavities where absorption into the blood is unlikely; also used as an enema.
- sterile water, USP—must be labeled NOT FOR INJECTION.

EPIDURALS

An epidural is a type of CSP usually used in connection with surgery or childbirth. The epidural is injected intrathecally (next to the spine) to help control pain. An individual epidural may be a combination of a narcotic and an anesthetic, or just an anesthetic. Since the epidural is injected intrathecally, this CSP must be preservative-free.

INJECTABLE PELLETS OR IMPLANTS

Injectable pellets are small, sterile, cylinders that are implanted under the skin to provide continuous release of a medication over a certain span of time. They are usually placed under the skin at the thigh or abdomen by using a special injecting device or by surgical incision. Pellets generally contain powerful doses of a hormone. Some examples of hormones that can be administered as an injectable pellet include:

- estradiol—one of the sex hormones
- testosterone—one of the sex hormones
- deoxycorticosterone—a steroid hormone produced by the adrenal gland
- levonorgestrel (contraceptive)—a birth control drug

INSULIN

Insulin is a hormone produced naturally by the body. The function of insulin is to take up glucose (sugar) from the blood and store it as glycogen. Patients with the disease **diabetes mellitus** do not produce enough insulin. As a result, blood sugar levels rise. Ideally, the blood glucose level should be between 70 and 140 mg/dL. In diabetes, abnormally high blood sugar levels can produce blurred vision, frequent urination, increased thirst, and weight loss.

To make up for the low or nonexistent insulin levels, insulin injections and/or dietary changes are used. In mild cases of diabetes, insulin medication is sometimes effective.

Syringes and Potency

In earlier chapters, you learned that dosage is measured in milliliters (mL). The potency of all insulin injections is expressed in USP insulin units per milliliter. For example, 100 units of insulin means there are 100 active units of insulin in each milliliter of liquid in solution. So you can see that a 100 unit insulin syringe contains a more potent dose of insulin than a 50 unit syringe.

All insulin injections show the expiration date, which must not be more than 24 months after the manufacture date. In addition, packages are color-coded according to strength. This helps avoid confusing one insulin dose with another.

An important job of the pharmacist is to make sure a physician's written insulin orders are read correctly when preparing an insulin injection. As you can probably imagine, misreading an order for 6 U of insulin and preparing instead a 60 U injection could have serious consequences.

Insulin syringes come in 30 unit, 50 unit and 100 unit sizes. The needles are very short and very fine. An insulin syringe would not be useful in preparing a CSP because of the different calibrations and the length and fineness of the needle.

Proper Administration

Insulin is usually administered by injection. However, in mild cases of diabetes, a combination of oral medication, dietary changes, and increased exercise may also be effective. In the case of injected insulin, it is important that patients remember to rotate the injection site. Failure to do so can result in a buildup of fibrous tissue at the injection site.

It is also important to allow the insulin to come to room temperature before injecting. Repeatedly injecting cold insulin can create an indentation in the tissue at the injection site.

Types of Insulin

A specific type of insulin preparation is needed for each patient. The two most critical characteristics of any insulin preparation are:

- Action—how long it takes the insulin to take effect in the body
- Duration—how long the insulin remains effective in the body

There are several types of insulin used for injection, each with its own characteristics. Some of these are described below. Some, but not all, of these individual insulin preparations can be mixed together to achieve the specific action and duration of insulin needed by the patient.

- Insulin injection—a sterile water-based solution; commonly prepared from cow or pig pancreas, or both; contains 100 or 500 USP insulin units per milliliter; colorless to straw-colored, depending on the potency (a 500 U injection is straw-colored)
- Human Insulin—**Humulin**; first available in 1983; cultured from a non-disease-forming strain of *E. coli* using DNA that codes for human insulin; one type is fast-acting with a short duration; the other type is medium-acting with a long duration
- Lispro Insulin—consists of zinc insulin lispro crystals in a water-based solution; shorter acting than regular insulin

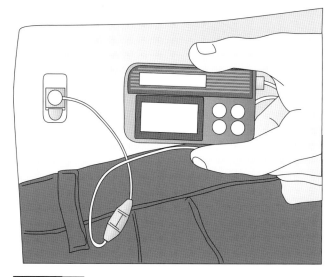

FIGURE 8-2 Today's insulin pumps are lightweight, but expensive.

■ Insulin Aspart—uses baker's yeast to produce insulin; similar acting to lispro insulin
■ Isophane Insulin suspension (NPH Insulin)—prepared from zinc insulin crystals and protamine (obtained from the sperm or mature testes of a specific group of fish); medium-acting; commonly used as an insulin replacement
■ Insulin Glargine—a long duration insulin product designed for daily injections at bedtime
■ Extended Insulin Zinc Suspension—a sterile suspension of zinc insulin crystals in a water-based solution with sodium acetate; long duration

Insulin Pumps

An alternative to injecting insulin is using a pump. **Insulin pumps** are designed to keep blood glucose levels within a normal range. Early insulin pumps were large and cumbersome. It wasn't until the mid-1980s that small, portable pumps were invented. Today's insulin pumps are lightweight, but expensive (Fig. 8-2).

How Insulin Pumps Work

Today's insulin pumps are much smaller and lighter than earlier models. The pump reservoir holds about 300 U of U-100 insulin. A computer chip in the pump makes it easy for the patient to program the amount of insulin to be released. The infusion set is usually inserted subcutaneously into the abdomen, where the insulin is quickly absorbed. Of course, the insertion site must be kept clean to prevent infection.

T I P Swabbing the insertion site regularly with IPA or a similar cleaning agent is an easy way to prevent infection.

NASAL PREPARATIONS

Nasal preparations are water-based solutions that are sprayed into the nose to help treat rhinitis. **Rhinitis** is the irritation and inflammation of the internal areas of the nose. The most common symptom of rhinitis is a runny nose. This condition can be caused by viruses, bacteria, or irritants. Usually during rhinitis, large amounts of mucus and congestion are produced. Examples of nasal preparations are:

■ nose drops
■ nose sprays
■ nose jellies
■ nasal inhalers

According to the FDA, all nasal preparations should be sterile when dispensed. Some nasal solutions may contain buffers, preservatives, and other additives. Because of the delicate cilia inside the nasal passageways, nasal solutions must also be isotonic.

Proper Administration

As a pharmacy technician, remind patients how important it is to prevent contamination of all nasal preparations. Tell patients that the nasal product is to be used by only one person. For the proper administration of nasal drops or nasal sprays, patients should follow the instructions given on the package or by the pharmacist.

Compounding Considerations

Compounded nasal solutions must be sterilized before dispensing. To do this, a bacterial filter and sterile container are used in a laminar airflow hood or compounding aseptic isolator. An autoclave may also be used for steam sterilization once the product is compounded. However, make sure that the drugs used in the product are not affected by the high temperature and pressure of the autoclave or by the bacterial filter.

OPHTHALMICS

Ophthalmic solutions and suspensions are sterile, particle-free products administered in the eye. Most are water-based or sterile, isotonic, sodium-chloride-based. Like nasal preparations, ophthalmics may also contain buffers, preservatives, antioxidants, and other additives and agents. Also like nasal preparations, the delicate membranes of the eye make isotonicity a requirement.

Compounding Requirements

Ophthalmic solutions are sterile and particle-free. To accomplish this, compounding must take place in a sterile environment such as a laminar airflow hood or compounding aseptic isolator, and, of course, using aseptic technique.

Sterility and Preservation

Ophthalmic solutions and suspensions may be sterilized in one of two ways:

- using an autoclave
- using a bacterial filter

Autoclaving is a more efficient way to achieve sterilization. But the high temperatures produced inside the autoclave may have a negative effect on the solution or suspension. Bacterial filters are an acceptable alternative since they do not rely on heat or high pressure. Another advantage bacterial filters have over autoclaving is that filters remove all particles (including dust and fibers) from the solution or suspension (Fig. 8-3).

To help ensure sterility once the ophthalmic is being used, preservatives may be added during compounding.

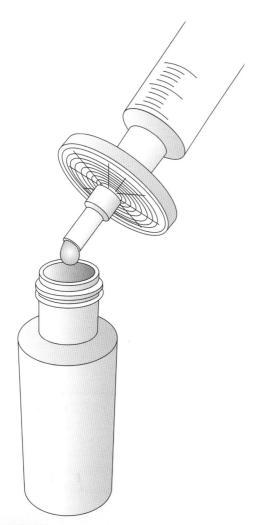

FIGURE 8-3 Bacterial filter for ophthalmic solutions and suspensions.

Because certain situations or patients may not be able to tolerate preservatives, preservative-free ophthalmics are also made.

Isotonicity

The tonicity of ophthalmic solutions should be close to that of tears. This is an amount close to a 0.9% NaCl solution. The tonicity range of ophthalmics ranges from 0.6% to 2% NaCl. Ophthalmics must also be chemically and physically stable, and free of allergy-causing agents or chemicals.

Buffering

Remember that the pH of a solution describes how acidic or alkaline the solution is. The pH of an ophthalmic and the pH of the fluid in the eye must be compatible. This is a pH of about 7.4. If the pH of the ophthalmic is not compatible with the fluid in the eye, irritation may result, or the product may become unstable. To obtain the desired pH of an ophthalmic, a **buffer** is often added to the ophthalmic product. Commonly used buffers for ophthalmics are monobasic sodium phosphate solution and dibasic sodium phosphate solution.

Viscosity and Thickening Agents

The **viscosity** of a fluid describes how quickly the fluid is able to flow. The slower the ophthalmic flows, the longer it is exposed to body tissues, and the greater the effect of the product. When compounding ophthalmics, a thickening agent is often added to increase the viscosity of the product. A common thickening agent used for this purpose is methylcellulose.

Bioavailability

Another important characteristic of ophthalmics is bioavailability. This describes the amount of the product that actually reaches the eye tissue. In other words, the greater the bioavailability of an ophthalmic, the more effective it is. Several factors affect the bioavailability of ophthalmics:

- protein-binding-when an ophthalmic is administered, proteins in the eye fluid may bind with the drug and decrease its effectiveness.
- tears—enzymes in tears may degrade certain drug substances

Packaging

Most ophthalmics are packaged in soft plastic containers with a fixed built-in dropper. This type of packaging helps protect it from contamination and makes administration easier.

Proper Administration

Since ophthalmic solutions and suspensions are sterile products, they should be clear and free of any cloudiness

PROCEDURE

How To Use Eye Drops

1. Wash your hands with soap and warm water.
2. Lie on your back or turn your face upward.
3. Pull down and pinch the lower lid to create a pocket.
4. Being careful not to touch the dropper to the eye, put one drop in the eye.
5. Release the lid, close and the eye and look around.
6. If additional drops are needed, repeat step 5 above.
7. Replace the cap on the bottle.

PROCEDURE

How To Use Ear Drops

1. Wash your hands with soap and warm water.
2. Use the medicine dropper to draw up a small amount of ear drop solution.
3. Lie on your side so that the affected ear faces toward the ceiling.
4. Position the tip of the dropper so that it is just inside the ear canal. Do not touch the dropper against the ear or any other object. Hold the earlobe up and back for adults. Hold the earlobe down and back for children.
5. Squeeze the prescribed number of drops into the ear canal. Allow the drops to flow into the ear canal.
6. Remain lying down for 3-5 minutes.
7. Prevent any liquid from leaking out of the ear canal by using a clean piece of cotton. Bring the head upright.
8. Replace the cap on the bottle.

or particulate matter. Before administering ophthalmic solutions or suspensions, the hands should be washed thoroughly. Suspensions should be shaken. Care should be taken not to touch the eye, as that action will contaminate the tip of the applicator. Remove and replace the cap of an eye drop container immediately before and after use.

OTIC PREPARATIONS

Otic preparations are products that are used in the ear. Most otic preparations are solutions, but ointments and suspensions are also used sometimes. Even though otic preparations are compounded in a sterile environment using aseptic technique, they are not considered sterile medications. This is because they are administered externally.

Proper Administration

Your job as pharmacy technician is to make sure patients administer otic preparations correctly. Be sure to explain to patients that the otic preparation is for use in the ear only, that suspensions need to be shaken, and that solutions should be warmed in the hands before use.

PEDIATRIC PREPARATIONS

Newborn babies and pediatric patients (children) may need medicines like antibiotics, antifungals, antivirals, narcotics, and insulin as well. But because their liver, kidneys and other organs are still developing, these young patients require that their medications be diluted before being administered. For the same reason, pediatric and newborn dilutions and preparations must also be preservative-free.

A **dilution** is a process that makes a more concentrated substance less concentrated. For example, let's say you have a stock of 100 U/mL insulin. But the dose of insulin

ordered for a newborn is 5 U. The actual amount of insulin needed for a dose of 5 U would be 0.05 mL of the 100 U/mL stock solution. But such a small amount would be very difficult to measure accurately. However, if the 100 mL insulin stock is diluted to 10 U/mL, then the 5 U is more easily measured as 0.5 mL.

PATIENT CONTROLLED ANALGESIA

For patients suffering from acute or chronic patient-controlled analgesia (PCA) offers gre These units are ideal for patients experien from surgery, labor, a sickle cell crisis, a Developed in the late 1980s, this pump-ba allows patients to self-administer their pres medication. The biggest advantage of PCA he vides a constant level of pain relief as op inject-as-needed method.

How the Pump Works

A typical PCA pump includes a syringe or c essed ing the drug, and a programmable unit. to the by the patient, releases a specific amoun h care patient's system. The pump can be load professional, or filled with preloaded c

PROTEINS

SP that is
Special protein preparations are other CSPs
sometimes ordered for a patient. I

discussed in this chapter, these are also compounded aseptically. Due to their sticky nature, proteins cannot be filtered during the compounding process. As the particles stick to the filter, the strength of the preparation is decreased.

Types

There are several types of protein preparations. They include:

- albumin—used to treat hypovolemic shock, newborn liver dysfunction, and other conditions; dispose of empty albumin vials only in an approved sharps container
- plasma protein fraction (PPF)—sterile solution used as a single-IV-dose to prevent and treat hypovolemic shock and cases of kidney dysfunction
- immunoglobulin (GAMMAR, IgG)—a sterile single-dose preparation used to help weakened immune systems return to normal; chemo gloves should be worn when preparing IgG; a IgG product must be carefully reconstituted according to instruction before being administered
- Factor VIII (ALPHANATE)—a sterile, single-dose concentrate of antihemophilic factor (AHF) used to prevent and control bleeding in patients with hemophilia; chemo gloves should be worn when preparing Factor VIII; ordered in units; store in refrigerator; bring to room temperature before administering; extremely expensive
- Factor IX (KONYNE)—sterile, single-dose concentrate of AHF used for IV administration; handling and other procedures are the same as those for Factor VIII

dling

preparations should never be used if they cloudy or turbid or if there is sediment in the vial.

PARENTERAL NUTRITION

solutions are solutions injected through the mbrane directly into a blood vessel, muscle, other tissue. When a patient is not able to ugh nutrition through the mouth, a physorder a total parenteral nutrition (TPN) ve administered to patients directly into a ad over a 10-12 hour period. Since TPNs are and intravenously, these CSPs must be sterile trat ed aseptically. The IV route of adminis- in th through a central line (through a vein bdomen) or a peripheral line (through

a vein not in the chest or abdomen). TPN solutions contain:

- proteins
- fats
- sugars
- water
- minerals
- electrolytes
- vitamins in liquid form

TPN bags are compounded on a daily basis according to the specific needs of the patient. The bags range in size from 100 mL to 3000 mL.

Ingredients

The basic ingredients in a TPN bag are dextrose (the major source of calories), amino acids (required for protein synthesis), fat (to supply essential fatty acids), basic electrolytes (Na, K, Mg, Ca, and P), vitamins, trace elements (Cu, Cr, Zn, Mn, Se), and histamine H_2-receptor antagonists (prevents and treats upper gastrointestinal ulcers).

Types

There are two basic types of TPN formulas—the "3-in-1" and the "2-in-1". The most complete is the "all–in-one" or "3-in-1" TPN formula which contains amino acids, carbohydrates, and lipids (fats) in the same container. The "2-in-1" formula contains no lipids because they are hung separately.

The advantage of a "3-in-1" is that everything is contained in one bag. However, because the lipids are white and opaque, it is difficult to see any particulate matter than may be in the TPN. The advantage of a "2-in-1" is that the lipids are separate leaving you with a clear bag that can easily be inspected for particulate matter. Each facility will have a policy of which type they use.

Nutrient and Fluid Requirements

The general 24-hour nutrient and fluid requirements for an average adult receiving TPN are:

- Fluids—2,500-3,500 mL or 500-2,000 mL for an adult in kidney failure
- Protein—0.8 to 2.0 g protein per kilogram of actual body weight (ABW)
- Dextrose—302-5-4 g/day for a 70 kg adult
- IV Fat Emulsion—given as 1, 2, or 3 kcal/mL; IV fat should make up 1-4% of the total calories

Fluid, Electrolytes and Minerals

The first step in ordering a TPN is deciding the total volume of the product. The physician does this by using the patient's body weight or body surface area.

The basic additives commonly used in a TPN may be:

- amino acids 10%, trophamine 6%
- dextrose 70%, dextrose 50%
- sterile water
- lipids—10%, 20%, or 30%

The electrolytes and minerals added to the base solution include sodium, potassium, chloride, phosphate, calcium, and magnesium. The functions of daily electrolytes and minerals in TPN are described below.

- sodium—determines total body water
- potassium—contributes to nerve and muscle function; regulates water balance in cells
- chloride—regulates water balance inside and outside cells; helps maintain proper blood volume, blood pressure, and pH of body fluids
- calcium—helps many body functions; needed for proper bone formation and maintenance, nerve function, muscle contraction, blood clotting, and heart function
- magnesium—needed for muscular and nervous system
- phosphate—used for bone growth, energy, fighting infection, and muscle function

Calcium and Phosphate

The amount of calcium and phosphate added to a TPN mixture is critical. If not added in the correct order, in the correct amounts, and/or at the correct temperature, a solid mass called a precipitate forms which can block the flow of the TPN. A **precipitate** is a solid mass that forms in a solution when two or more substances react. To prevent the formation of a calcium phosphate precipitate in a TPN admixture, the FDA has recommended the following precautions:

- The solubility of calcium should be calculated based on the TPN volume at the time the calcium is added—NOT on the final TPN volume.
- When calcium and phosphate are added to a TPN admixture, the phosphate should be added first.
- When calculating the concentration of phosphate additives, the volume of the TPN at the time the phosphate is added should be considered—NOT the final TPN volume.
- The IV line should be flushed between the addition of any ingredients or additives that may be incompatible.
- Consider administering calcium separately.
- Admixtures should be checked during the compounding process for precipitate formation.
- Use a filter when infusing TPN admixtures.

Amino Acids

Amino acids are the molecular building blocks of proteins. Proteins play a role in many body functions. Amino acids are also a source of nitrogen, which the body needs to utilize proteins.

Some amino acids are called **essential amino acids** because the body does not produce them. It is therefore *essential* that these amino acids be supplied through the diet. Nonessential amino acids, on the other hand, are made naturally by the body.

Automated Compounding Devices

Some TPN admixtures may contain 50 or more individual components. Compounding TPN formulas by hand requires great precision and lots of time. One option for completing this labor-intensive task is to use an automated compounding device (ACD.) An ACD is a programmable, computerized device that delivers nutrients in a pre-determined sequence.

ACD devices are available for use with large-volume solutions or with small-volume solutions.

Sample Order

Each TPN begins with a physician's order. The order is then sent to the pharmacy to be compounded. A hospital may have a standardized TPN order, designed for the average patient. The physician can specify how a TPN order differs from this standardized order.

The order must take into consideration whether the TPN is to be administered through a central line or a peripheral line. The factors that determine this are:

- the type of medication being administered
- the osmolarity and pH of the TPN solution
- duration of therapy
- diagnosis or medical condition of the patient
- patient preferences
- current availability and condition of patient's veins
- patient history
- secondary risk factors

A sample TPN order is shown in Table 8-1.

CHAPTER HIGHLIGHTS

- CSPs include products such as biologics, hazardous drugs, radiopharmaceuticals, insulin, chemotherapy agents, insulin, injectable pellets, irrigations, nasal preparations, epidurals, ophthalmics, otic preparations, pediatric preparations, patient-controlled analgesics, proteins, and total parenteral nutrition products.

TABLE 8-1   Sample TPN Order

Patient Name: GD
Age: 52   Height: 6'1"   Weight (ABW*):   IBW: 80 kg
                                       176 lb, 80 kg

AVERAGE 24-HOUR ADULT REQUIREMENTS FOR TPN COMPONENTS

Component	Requirement	Amount Ordered	Evaluation
Fluid	30-35 mL/kg	30 mL/kg	OK
Protein (AA*)	0.8-2.0 g AA/kg ABW	1.5 AA/kg ABW	OK
Dextrose	3-5 mg/kg/min	3 mg/kg/min	OK
IV lipid	≤≤30% of total kcal	23%	OK
kcal/kg ABW	25-35 kcal/kg ABW	26.9 kcal/kg ABW	OK
Sodium	1-2 mEq/kg ABW	1.9 mEq/kg	OK
Potassium	1-2 mEq/kg ABW	1 mEq/kg	OK
Phosphate	20-40 mmol	30 mmol	OK
Magnesium	8-20 mEq	24 mEq	OK
Calcium	10-15 mEq	10 mEq	OK
Trace elements	3 mL	3 mL	OK
Vitamins	10 mL unit	10-mL unit	OK

*ABW is actual body weight; AA is amino acids.
(Table reprinted from Thompson JE. *A Practical Guide to Contemporary Pharmacy Practice.* 3rd ed. Baltimore, MD: Wolters Kluwer Health/Lippincott Williams & Wilkins, 2009.)

- A hazardous drug is a drug that can cause serious effects such as cancer, organ toxicity, fertility problems, genetic damage, or birth defects.
- The equipment needed to compound a hazardous drug CSP includes closed system transfer devices, a BSC (biological safety cabinet) or CACI (compounding aseptic containment isolator), and chemotherapy gloves.
- Hazardous drugs must be compounded in at least an ISO Class 5 environment.
- The safest method for manipulating hazardous drugs in a BSC or CACI is to use a closed system transfer device (CSTD).
- The environmental requirements and standards for compounding radiopharmaceuticals include using shielded vials and/or syringes such as those in a CSTD, and working in a certified ISO Class 5 environment located in an ISO Class 8 (no more than 100,000 particles per cubic foot) air environment.
- When a patient is not able to receive enough nutrition through the mouth, a physician may order a total parenteral nutrition (TPN) bag.
- The basic fluid components in a TPN are amino acids 10%, trophamine 6%, dextrose 70%, dextrose 50%, sterile water, and lipids—10%, 20%, or 30%. The electrolytes and minerals that may be added to the TPN include: sodium, potassium, chloride, calcium, magnesium, and phosphorous.
- Types of automated compounding devices include the Nutrimix Macro TPN Compounder for large volume solutions or the Nutrimix Micro TPN Compounder for small volume solutions.

QUICK QUIZ

Answer the following multiple-choice questions.

1. Which of the following groups is not a source for some biologic CSPs?
   a. amino acids
   b. vitamins
   c. hormones
   d. antibiotics
2. Which body system is most affected by a vaccination?
   a. reproductive system
   b. nervous system
   c. digestive system
   d. immune system
3. Cancer, organ toxicity, fertility problems, genetic damage, or birth defects may be caused by
   a. vaccinations
   b. otic preparations
   c. hazardous drugs
   d. immunizations

4. A large chemo spill is considered anything over
   a. 5 mL
   b. 5 dL
   c. 5 U
   d. 5 oz
5. What does TPN stand for?
   a. total primary nutrition
   b. total parenteral naturalism
   c. total parental nutrition
   d. total parenteral nutrition

Please answer each of the following questions in one to three sentences.

1. Why must a TPN be sterile or prepared aseptically?

   _____

   _____

2. What is PCA and what is the advantage to using it?

   _____

   _____

3. Why are dilutions necessary for pediatric preparations?

   _____

   _____

4. Why is the correct addition of calcium and phosphorous to TPN admixtures so critical?

   _____

   _____

5. How is an insulin syringe different from a syringe you would use to prepare a CSP??

   _____

   _____

Answer the following questions as either true or false.

1. ____ Chemotherapy drugs are only used to treat cancer.
2. ____ Malignant cells refer only to cancerous cells.
3. ____ Otic solutions should be prepared in a laminar airflow workbench because they are considered sterile preparations.
4. ____ A newborn receiving an injection could receive either a preservative-free preparation or a preparation that contains a preservative.
5. ____ A "3-in-1" TPN contains the amino acids, carbohydrates and lipids all in one container.

Match the term in the left column with the correct description from the right column.

1. buffer
2. cold chain
3. PhaSeal
4. viscosity
5. technetium-99m

a. how a fluid is able to flow
b. the steps taken to keep a biologic at a specific low temperature
c. isotope used in radiopharmaceuticals
d. A CSTD that keeps human exposure to chemotherapy drugs to a minimum
e. used to obtain a desired pH

CHAPTER 9

Quality Assurance

- Evaluate the training requirements for personnel compounding CSPs.
- Determine the media-fill testing performed by personnel compounding CSPs.
- Identify various commonly used methods of sterilization.
- Describe how to perform visual and physical inspections of a CSP in various storage devices.
- Examine the need for compounding accuracy and ensuring that a CSP has been compounded correctly.
- Evaluate the criteria for sterility and pyrogen testing.
- Identify the methods for completing sterility and pyrogen testing.

KEY TERMS

filtration—the passage of a fluid or solution through a sterilizing grade membrane to produce a sterile effluent

media-fill test—a test used to qualify the aseptic technique of compounding personnel or processes, and to ensure that the processes used produce a sterile product that is without microbial contamination

product—a commercially manufactured sterile drug that has been evaluated for safety and efficacy by the U.S. Food and Drug Administration

pyrogen—a fever-producing organic substance arising from microbial contamination

quality assurance—the set of activities used to ensure that the procedures used in the preparation of sterile products lead to products that meet predetermined standards of quality

sterilization—the destruction of all living organisms and their spores, or their complete removal from a preparation

Quality assurance is the foundation for all compounded sterile preparations. Without it, patients, pharmacists, technicians, and the public at large are placed at risk. Because of the differing risk levels that you've learned about previously, the steps taken to ensure absolute sterility vary in process and procedure. However, the compounding, storage, and delivery of sterile products are all subject to stringent oversight and guidelines. If these guidelines are not followed, contamination, in some form, is certain to occur.

By studying this chapter, you will be able to identify the rigorous training requirements that all personnel who come into contact with sterile products must undergo. You will learn the procedures for media-fill testing and for various methods of sterilization. You will also be able to follow the steps for visual and physical inspections of sterile products. Finally, you will evaluate the criteria for sterility and pyrogen testing,

and learn the proper methods for completing these tests.

OVERVIEW OF QUALITY ASSURANCE PROGRAM

The United States Pharmacopeia (USP)'s Chapter 797 (USP <797>) has provided clear, specific, and enforceable standards for **quality assurance** in the preparation of sterile products. Their goal is for every CSP provider to have a formal quality assurance program in place. This program should monitor, evaluate, correct, and improve the activities and processes used to compound sterile preparations. The USP also encourages conducting regular follow-ups to ensure that if problems do occur, proper procedures are being followed.

The USP <797> suggests that quality assurance programs consist of the following components:

- Formalization of program policies in writing
- Consideration of all aspects of the preparation and dispensing of products
- Description of monitoring and evaluation activities
- Specification of how results are reported and evaluated
- Identification of follow-up mechanisms that can be used when procedural problems are noted
- Description of the individuals responsible for each aspect of the quality assurance program

The key to establishing a good quality assurance plan is to have objectives, which are measurable indicators for monitoring processes and activities that are particularly high-risk, high-volume, or problem-prone. It's important for the quality assurance program to be evaluated on an annual basis to ensure that it is comprehensive and up-to-date.

COMPOUNDING PERSONNEL

The compounding personnel are the first-line defenders of quality assurance. Their responsibilities are many and vary from person to person. In general, however, they are responsible for making sure of the following:

- CSPs are accurately identified, measured, diluted, and mixed
- CSPs are correctly prepared, sterilized, packaged, sealed, labeled, stored, dispensed, and distributed
- appropriate cleanliness conditions are being maintained
- labeling and supplementary instructions are provided for the proper clinical administration of CSPs

Compounding personnel are trained in an appropriate and systematic manner so that they can competently fulfill all of these responsibilities.

Training

A written quality assurance procedure is the first step in any worthwhile training program. Expert compounding personnel oversee the training, which may include audio-video instructional sources and professional publications on aseptic manipulations and maintaining an ISO Class 5 environment. The quality assurance procedure should include the following checks applied to specific CSPs:

- accuracy and precision of measuring and weighing
- sterility requirements
- sterilization and purification methods

- safe limits and ranges for strengths of ingredients, bacterial endotoxins, and particulate matter
- the pH level of the CSP
- labeling accuracy and completeness
- beyond-use date assignment
- packaging and storage requirements

As part of the training program in aseptic manipulation skills, compounding personnel must perform a didactic review of the skills required and pass a written test of their knowledge. After initial validation, they must also retake and pass these examinations either annually (for low- and medium-risk compounding) or semiannually (for high-risk compounding).

For those who prepare hazardous drugs, their training includes didactic overview of hazardous drugs, including mutagenic, teratogenic, and carcinogenic properties. Ongoing training continues when new hazardous drugs are introduced into the marketplace. At the very least, a hazardous drug training must include:

- safe aseptic manipulation practices
- negative pressure techniques to use when working with a biological safety cabinet or compounding aseptic containment isolators
- correct use of closed-system vial-transfer devices
- containment, cleanup, and disposal procedures for breakages and spills
- treatment of personal contact and inhalation exposure

In addition to a written demonstration of their knowledge, compounding personnel must pass hands-on evaluations to ensure that they can put their knowledge into practice. Some of these evaluations include:

- skill assessments using observational audit tools
- media-fill testing
- hand hygiene practices
- garbing practices
- cleaning and disinfection procedures

Compounding personnel who fail their assessments are immediately reinstructed and re-evaluated by expert compounding personnel to ensure that they are brought up to an acceptable level of functioning.

Competency Evaluations

Part of the hands-on evaluations that personnel must undergo includes the assessment of competencies in garbing, hand washing, and gloved-fingertip sampling procedures, procedures which have been described thoroughly in previous chapters. Mastery of these competencies is crucial to ensuring that aseptic manipulations are conducted in the most sterile, controlled environment. The chance of contaminating a low- or medium-risk CSPs depends greatly on hand hygiene and garbing practices.

Garbing and Hand washing

Garbing and hand washing procedures are evaluated via visual inspection by a supervising authority. The outcomes are documented and maintained to provide a permanent record for long-term assessment of competency. USP <797> suggests that personnel be evaluated on the basis of the following criteria:

- Presents in a clean, appropriate attire and manner
- Wears no cosmetics or jewelry upon entry into ante-areas
- Brings no food or drink into or stored in ante-areas or buffer areas
- Is aware of the line of demarcation separating clean and dirty sides and observes required activities
- Dons shoe covers or designated clean-area shoes one at a time, placing the covered or clean shoe on the clean side of the line of demarcation
- Dons beard cover if necessary
- Dons head cover, assuming all hair is covered
- Dons face mask to cover bridge of nose down to and including the chin
- Performs hand hygiene procedure by wetting hands and forearms and washing using soap and warm water for at least 30 seconds
- Dries hands and forearms using a lint-free towel or hand dryer
- Selects the appropriately sized gown and examines for holes, tears, or other defects
- Dons gown and ensures full closure
- Disinfects hands again using a waterless, alcohol-based surgical hand scrub with persistent activity and allows hands to dry thoroughly before donning sterile gloves
- Dons appropriate-sized sterile gloves, ensuring a tight fit with no excess glove material at fingertips
- Examines gloves for any tears, holes, or other defects
- While engaging in sterile compounding activities, routinely disinfects gloves with sterile 70% isopropyl alcohol before working in the direct compounding area and after touching items or surfaces that may contaminate gloves

Once the compounding personnel have successfully engaged in compounding in a sterile environment, they are evaluated on their exit procedures. These include whether they:

- Remove personal protective equipment on the clean side of the ante-area
- Remove gloves and performs hand hygiene
- Remove gown and discard it, or hang it on a hook if it is to be reused the same work day
- Remove and discard mask, head cover, and beard cover (if used)

- Remove shoe cover or shoe one at a time, ensuring that the uncovered foot is on the dirty side of the line of demarcation (this must happen every time they exit the compounding area)

T I P Remember to keep the contaminated foot on the proper side of the line of demarcation when donning shoe covers or clean-area shoes. After completing the compounding procedure, remove the shoe cover or clean-shoe one foot at a time, placing the uncovered foot over the line of demarcation.

Gloved Fingertip Sampling

Compounding personnel undergo gloved fingertip sampling to determine their competency in garbing and hand washing. Sterile agar plates are used to test their gloved fingertips and assess the adequacy of aseptic work practices. Before they are allowed to prepare CSPs, compounding personnel must successfully complete an initial competency evaluation and gloved fingertip/thumb sampling procedure (resulting in 0 colony-forming units found) at least three times.

To complete the sampling, compounding personnel supply a gloved fingertip and thumb sample from each hand by pressing each finger and thumb onto agar plates. The plates are incubated for the appropriate time and temperature. It is important to note that immediately before sampling, the gloves should NOT be disinfected with 70% sterile IPA, which would provide false-negative results.

Once the samples have been taken, the gloves are removed, and hand hygiene procedures are followed. The results of the agar-plate testing are reported as the number of colony-forming units per employee per hand. Depending on the outcome, personnel may require additional training and testing.

The gloved-fingertip test is conducted at least annually for those who compound low- and medium-risk CSPs and semiannually for those who compound high-risk CSPs using one or more sample collections during any media-fill test procedure.

Media-Fill Testing

Media-fill testing is used to assess the aseptic skills of compounding personnel. This test replicates the most challenging and stressful conditions actually encountered when preparing particular risk-level CSPs or sterilizing high-risk CSPs. Depending on whether low- and medium-risk or high-risk CSPs are being prepared, re-evaluation occurs either annually or semiannually, respectively. Once begun, this test cannot be interrupted.

During a media-fill test, a commercially available sterile fluid culture medium (such as Soybean-Casein Digest Medium), which is used to promote exponential colonization of the bacteria that are most likely to be transmitted to CSPs from the compounding personnel and environment, is substituted for the actual drug product to simulate admixture compounding. Depending on the risk level, the steps in this test may vary.

For low-risk CSP media-fill testing, the following steps might be taken

1. Within an ISO Class 5 air quality environment, transfer three sets of four 5-mL aliquots of medium with the same sterile 10-mL syringe and vented needle combination into separate sealed, empty sterile 30-mL clear vials.
2. Aseptically affix sterile adhesive seals to the rubber closures on the three filled vials.
3. Incubate the vials at 20-25°C or 30-35°C for at least 14 days.
4. If two temperatures are used, incubate the containers for at least 7 days at each temperature.
5. Inspect for microbial growth over 14 days.

For medium-risk CSP media-fill testing, the following steps might be taken:

1. Within an ISO Class 5 air quality environment, transfer six 100-mL aliquots of medium by gravity through separate tubing sets into separate evacuated sterile containers.
2. Arrange the six containers as three pairs.
3. Exchange two 5-mL aliquots from one container to the other container in the pair using a sterile 10-mL syringe and 18-gauge needle combination.
4. After adding a 5-mL aliquot from the first container to the second container in the pair, agitate the second container for 10 seconds, and then remove a 5-mL aliquot and return it to the first container in the pair.
5. Agitate the first container for 10 seconds.
6. Transfer the next 5-mL aliquot from the first container back to the second container in the pair.
7. After the two 5-mL aliquot exchanges in each pair of containers, aseptically inject a 5-mL aliquot of medium from each container into a sealed, empty, sterile 10-mL clear vial using a sterile 10-mL syringe and vented needle.
8. Affix sterile adhesive seals to the rubber closures on the three vials.
9. Incubate the vials at 20-25°C or 30-35°C for at least 14 days.
10. If two temperatures are used, incubate the containers for at least 7 days at each temperature.
11. Inspect for microbial growth over 14 days.

For high-risk CSP media-fill testing, the following steps might be taken

1. Dissolve 3 mL of medium in 100 mL of nonbacteriostatic water to make a 3% nonsterile solution.

PROCEED WITH CAUTION

Know Your Risk Level During Media-Fill Testing

There are considerable differences in media-fill testing procedures for low-, medium-, and high-risk CSPs. Once the media-fill testing begins, it can't be interrupted. Make sure you know the procedures for each risk type so that you can make the correct decisions during a media-fill test.

2. Draw 25 mL of the medium into each of three 30-mL sterile syringes. Transfer 5 mL from each syringe into separate sterile 10-mL vials (these are the positive controls to generate exponential microbial growth).
3. Under aseptic conditions and using aseptic techniques, affix a sterile 0.2- or 0.22-μm nominal pore-size filter unit and a 20-gauge needle to each syringe.
4. Inject the next 10 mL from each syringe into three separate 10-mL sterile vials. Repeat the process for three vials.
5. Label all vials.
6. Affix sterile adhesive seals to the closure of the nine vials.
7. Incubate the vials at 20-25°C or 30-35°C for at least 14 days.
8. If two temperatures are used, incubate the containers for at least 7 days at each temperature.
9. Inspect for microbial growth over 14 days.

Regardless of the CSP level, media-fill test failure results with visible turbidity in the medium on or before 14 days of incubation. Personnel whose media-fill test vials have one or more units showing visible microbial contamination are reinstructed and re-evaluated by expert compounding personnel to ensure that all aseptic work practice deficiencies are corrected.

STERILIZATION METHODS

Sterilization is the process of destroying all living organisms and their spores, or removing them completely from a pharmaceutical preparation. There are five general methods used for sterilizing pharmaceutical products:

1. steam
2. dry heat
3. filtration
4. gas
5. ionizing radiation

Typically, the licensed healthcare professionals who supervise compounding are responsible for selecting the appropriate method. USP <797> provides some general guidelines for matching CSPs and their components to the appropriate sterilization methods:

- CSPs should be able to maintain their physical and chemical stability when subjected to the selected sterilization method.
- Glass and metal devices may be covered tightly with aluminum foil and then exposed to dry heat in an oven at a mean temperature of 250°C for 30 minutes to achieve sterility and depyrogenation.
- Compounding personnel should determine from appropriate information sources that the sterile microporous membrane filter used to sterilize CSP solutions (during compounding or administration) is chemically and physically compatible with the CSP.

Steam Sterilization

Using steam to sterilize pharmaceutical preparations is an option if the product is able to physically withstand the procedure. It occurs in an autoclave and uses steam under pressure to produce the desired results.

Because it is impossible to increase the temperature of steam above 100°C under atmospheric conditions, pressure is used to achieve higher temperatures. However, it's important to note that it is the high temperature, *not* pressure, that destroys the microorganisms. Time, another factor in the destruction of microorganisms, has an inverse relationship with pressure, as you can see from the following list of pressure and times required for sterilization to occur:

- 10 lb of pressure (115.5°C or 240°F) for 30 minutes
- 15 lb of pressure (121.5°C or 250°F) for 20 minutes
- 20 lb of pressure (126.5°C or 260°F) for 15 minutes

As you can see, the greater the pressure, the higher the temperature achieved, and the less time required for sterilization.

For steam sterilization to be effective, the pharmaceutical preparations have to be able to withstand the heat and can be penetrated but not affected by moisture. Some of the best candidates for steam sterilization include:

- Solutions in ampules
- Sealed empty vials (containing a small amount of water)
- Bulk solutions
- Glassware
- Surgical dressings
- Instruments

Steam sterilization is not useful for:

- Oils
- Fats
- Oleaginous preparations
- Exposed powders
- Other preparations not penetrated by moisture

Dry Heat Sterilization

Dry heat sterilization is conducted in special ovens designed entirely for this purpose. These ovens can be powered by gas or electricity, and they're usually controlled by a thermostat.

Dry heat is less effective at killing microorganisms than moist heat, so the ovens must be fired for a longer time at a higher temperature. The parameters of the sterilization procedure are determined by the product's:

- Size
- Type
- Container heat distribution characteristics

To use the ovens optimally, the units to be sterilized should be as small as possible, and should not be crowded into the ovens. Rather, they should be positioned so that heated air can freely circulate throughout the chamber.

Dry heat sterilization usually takes place between 150° and 170°C for no less than 2 hours at a time. If a particular component melts at the higher end of that range, then a lower temperature is used for a longer period of time. On the other hand, if a chemical agent remains stable at 170°C, then it can be heated at the higher end of the range for a shorter time period. Dry heat is best used for substances that are not effectively sterilized by moist heat, such as:

- fixed oils
- glycerin
- petrolatum
- mineral oil
- paraffin
- zinc oxide or other heat-stable powders
- glassware
- surgical instruments
- packaging of dry powders
- packaging of nonaqueous solutions

Sterilization by Filtration

Filtration depends on the physical removal of microorganisms by adsorption on a filter medium or by a sieving mechanism. It is the best sterilization method for heat-sensitive solutions. The effectiveness of the filtered product can be greatly influenced by the microbial load in the solution being filtered, so any preparations sterilized in this manner must undergo stringent validation and monitoring.

Filters are commercially available and come with a variety of pore size specifications. The Millipore Corporation (based in Billerica, Massachusetts) produces a widely used filter known as the Millipore filter. This is a thin, plastic membrane composed of cellulosic esters with millions of pores per square inch. These pores make up about 80 percent of the membrane's volume, with the remainder composed of the filter material. Because of the high degree of porosity, the flow rates are much greater than those of other filters with the same particle retention capability.

Because Millipore filters are made from a variety of polymers, they're suitable for the filtration of almost any liquid or gas system. The filters come in a range of pore sizes, from 14 to 0.025 µm. The pore size is the main factor in the effective removal of microorganisms from a liquid, but other factors also come into play, including:

- electrical charge on the filter
- electrical charge of the microorganism
- pH of the solution
- temperature
- pressure or vacuum applied to the system

There are many advantages to bacterial filtration, including:

- its speed in the filtration of small quantities of solution
- its ability to sterilize thermolabile materials
- the inexpensive materials required
- the development and proliferation of membrane filter technology
- the complete removal of microorganisms, living and dead, and other particulate matter from a solution

One disadvantage to bacterial filtration is that, because the membrane is so fragile, it is critical to ensure that the assembly is properly secured and the membrane isn't ruptured or flawed during assembly, sterilization, or use. If the housing and filter assemblies are not first validated for compatibility and integrity, the entire sterilization process could be compromised. This is in stark contrast to dry and moist heat sterilization processes, which practically guarantee that sterilization occurs effectively. Another disadvantage is that filtering large quantities of liquid takes more time, especially if the liquid is viscous.

Generally, bacterial filtration is most appropriate when heat cannot be used or when only a small volume of liquid is being sterilized. Bacterial filtration is used conveniently and economically in community pharmacies for preparing sterile solutions such as ophthalmic solutions. The membrane filter is the most commonly used method in hospitals.

There has been some concern that membrane filters may also filter drug from a solution. However, current information suggests that little or no drug adsorption takes place during filtration with membrane filters. To err on the side of caution, refrain from filtering solutions containing small doses of drugs (<5 mg) until significant data demonstrate insignificant adsorption.

PROCEED WITH CAUTION

Pore Sizing and Membrane Placement

The preparation for membrane filtration poses the greatest risk of contamination during the procedure. Make sure that the housing and filter assemblies are validated for compatibility in advance of the procedure. This will help you to ensure that the procedure will run smoothly and the risk of contamination will be low.

Gas Sterilization

When you're dealing with heat-insensitive and moisture-sensitive materials, an optional method of sterilization is to expose them to ethylene oxide or propylene oxide gas. Although these gases are highly flammable when mixed with air, they can be used safely and effectively when diluted with carbon dioxide or a suitable fluorinated hydrocarbon. These mixtures are available commercially.

Sterilization with gas is enhanced and the exposure time required is reduced by increasing the relative humidity of the system to approximately 60 percent and increasing the temperature to 50°–60°C. If the moisture or temperature has to be decreased to accommodate for the limitations of the material being sterilized, then the exposure time increases. Sterilization with ethylene oxide gas requires about 4 to 16 hours of exposure.

One advantage of gas sterilization is its thorough penetrating qualities. It is especially useful in sterilizing:

- medical and surgical supplies
- catheters
- needles
- plastic disposable syringes in their final plastic packaging
- heat-labile enzyme preparations
- certain antibiotics

Some of the noteworthy disadvantages of gas sterilization include the fact that it requires the use of specialized equipment resembling an autoclave. Also, you must take greater precaution when using this method, because variables such as time, temperature, gas concentration, and humidity are not as firmly quantitated as in other methods of sterilization.

Sterilization by Ionizing Radiation

Ionizing radiation is probably the least used method of sterilization. The application of gamma rays and cathode rays to pharmaceutical preparations kills microorganisms effectively, but little is known about how it actually works.

One theory is that the rays alter the chemicals within or around the microorganism, forming deleterious new chemicals that are capable of destroying the cell. Another theory suggests that vital structures within the cell, such as the chromosomal nucleoprotein, are disoriented or destroyed by the radiation.

Regardless of what makes it happen, the cellular destruction radiation causes is complete and irreversible, which is advantageous. However, because highly specialized equipment is required, and because radiation may have other, unintended effects on products and their containers, this is an unpopular choice for sterilization.

PREPARATION RELEASE CHECKS AND TESTS

By this point, you have followed copious procedures, guidelines, and precautions in preparing a sterile product for distribution and use. It seems impossible that anything could have compromised the sterility of the product. However, there are still additional, final checks to be made before these CSPs can be released for administration.

First, you must visually examine CSPs that are intended to be made into solutions for the presence of particulate material, and do not administer them if such matter is observed. Also, before the CSPs are administered or dispensed, inspect the medication orders, written compounding procedure, preparation records, and expended materials used to make the CSPs for:

- accuracy of correct identities and amounts of ingredients
- aseptic mixing and sterilization
- packaging
- labeling
- expected physical appearance

Physical Inspection

Once CSP production has been completed, it is time to consult the written procedures for individually inspecting them. Some CSPs are not distributed immediately, so they must be inspected just before they leave the storage area, as described in the facility's written procedures.

Immediately after compounding, and as a condition of release, inspect each CSP unit (where possible) against lighted white or black, or both, backgrounds for evidence of visible particulates or other foreign matter. This inspection also includes conducting container-closure integrity testing and looking for any other apparent visual defects. It is best to squeeze the bag to make sure that it was not accidentally punctured during the compounding process. Squeezing and shaking the bag will also make sure that the drug is evenly distributed within the bag and not pooling at the point where it was injected.

Ensure that containers and seals are intact, and discard or segregate any CSPs with observed defects from acceptable products. When CSPs are not distributed promptly after preparation, conduct a predistribution inspection to ensure that a CSP with defects, such as cloudiness, precipitation, and leakage is not released. These defects can develop at any time between a product's release and distribution, so it's important to be alert when inspecting stored CSPs.

Inspection of a CSP must be done by someone other than the personnel who performed the initial compounding. This provides a neutral environment in which the CSP is inspected and considered by a fresh set of eyes, which reduces the probability of error.

Compounding Accuracy

Every facility has written procedures for double-checking compounding accuracy, and these procedures must be followed with every CSP preparation and before its release. This double check system includes:

- label accuracy
- accuracy of the addition of all drugs or ingredients used to prepare the finished product
- confirmation of the volumes and quantities of the finished product

Keep the used additive containers and the syringes used to measure the additive under quarantine with the final product until the final product check is completed. It may be policy for the volume to be checked prior to injection, especially for expensive medications. However, the policy may be for the volume to be checked after the process is complete. If this is the case, the plunger on the syringe should be pulled back to the same volume that was injected into the bag.

Compounding personnel should visually confirm that ingredients measured in syringes match the written order being compounded. Again, having a person other than the initial compounding personnel perform this check will ensure the credibility of the assessment.

One way to confirm the accuracy of measurements is by weighing a volume of the measured fluid. Then, calculate that volume by dividing the weight by the accurate value of the density, or specific gravity, of the measured fluid. Also, confirm the accuracy of the correct density values programmed into automated compounding devices before and after delivering volumes of the liquids assigned to each channel or port.

Using the following procedures to verify the correct identity and quality of CSPs before they are dispensed and administered:

1. Labels of CSPs bear the correct names and amounts of concentrations of ingredients, the total volume, the BUD, the appropriate route(s) of administration, the storage conditions, and other information for safe use.
2. There are correct identities, purities, and amounts of ingredients as determined by comparing the original written order with the written compounding record for the CSP.
3. The correct fill volumes in CSPs and correct quantities of filled units of the CSP have been obtained.

If the strength of the finished CSP cannot be confirmed to be accurate based on these three inspections, then assay the CSP using methods specific for the active ingredients.

Low- and medium-risk CSPs that exceed the USP <797> guidelines for beyond-use dating, described in an earlier chapter, must be tested according to USP Chapter <71> (Sterility Test). High-risk CSPs in groups of more than 25 must be tested according to USP chapters <71> (Sterility Test) and <85> (Bacterial Endotoxin Test).

Sterility Testing

High-risk CSPs that are prepared in groups of more than 25 identical individual single-dose packages (such as ampules, bags, syringes, or vials), are in multiple-dose vials, or are exposed for longer than 12 hours at 2°–8°C or 6 hours at 8°C or above before they are sterilized must meet the USP Chapter <71> sterility test before they are dispensed or administered. The membrane filtration method is the most compatible method for this type of testing.

On occasion, high-risk CSPs are dispensed before the results of their sterility tests are available. If this is the case, you must provide a written procedure recording daily observations of the incubating test specimens and immediate recall of the dispensed CSPs when there is any evidence of microbial growth in the test specimens. Also, you must notify the physician of a patient who may have received the potentially contaminated CSP to notify them of the potential risk.

Positive sterility test results require a rapid and systematic investigation of aseptic technique, environmental control, and other sterility assurance controls to identify the sources of contamination and correct problems in the methods and practices. Avoiding these outcomes altogether is ideal, but when contamination occurs, knowing the right steps to take is crucial to containing the problem.

TIP Don't forget that if a CSP is found to be contaminated after it's been released to a physician or health care worker, you must make every effort, without delay, to alert the personnel who are in possession of the product. Taking these actions in a timely fashion could save lives.

Pyrogen Testing

Pyrogens are fever-producing organic substances arising from microbial contamination and are responsible for many of the febrile reactions in patients who receive an injection. In these situations, it's believed that—although the injection underwent sterilization—a thermostable and water-soluble particle from bacteria or endotoxins remained in the water.

To sterilize the pyrogens from the water for injection, manufacturers commonly oxidize them, which changes the pyrogens to easily eliminated gases or nonvolatile solids that are easily separated from the water by fractional distillation. The oxidation agent of choice is potassium permanganate. The process occurs as follows:

- A small amount of barium hydroxide is added to potassium permanganate to impart alkalinity to the solution and produce nonvolatile barium salts.
- These reagents are added to water that has been distilled several times.
- Distillation is repeated.
- The chemical-free distillate is collected under aseptic conditions.
- Highly pure, sterile, and pyrogen-free water is the result.

PROCEDURE

Pyrogen Testing: Rabbit Test

1. Render the syringes, glassware, and needles free from pyrogens by heating at 250°C for no less than 30 minutes or by another suitable method.
2. Warm the product to be tested to 37 ± 2°C
3. Inject 10 mL per kilogram of body weight of the product into an ear vein in each of three rabbits, completing each injection within 10 minutes of the start of administration.
4. Record the rabbit body temperatures at 30-minute intervals 1 to 3 hours after the injection.
5. If no rabbit shows an individual increase in temperature of 0.5°C or more, the product meets the requirement for the absence of pyrogens.
6. If any rabbit shows an individual temperature increase of 0.5°C or more, continue the test using five other rabbits.
7. If not more than three of the eight rabbits show individual increases of 0.5°C or more, and if the sum of the eight individual maximal temperature increases does not exceed 3.3°C, the material under examination meets the requirements for the absence of pyrogens.

Once this process is complete, the official, USP-sanctioned pyrogen test must be performed to ensure that the pyrogens are absent.

Pyrogen Test

There are two procedures for pyrogen tests. One of them requires healthy rabbits that have been properly maintained in terms of diet, environment, and core body temperature. Their temperatures are used as the basis of whether a temperature increase results from the injection of a test solution. This procedure is described in the accompanying Procedure.

The other pyrogen test, known as the *Limulus* amebocyte lysate test (LAL), requires the use of an extract from the blood cells of the horseshoe crab (*Limulus polyphemus*), which contain an enzyme and protein system that coagulates in the presence of low levels of lipopolysaccharides. The USP Bacterial Endotoxins Test uses the LAL test and is considered to be more sensitive to endotoxin than the rabbit test. In fact, the Food and Drug Administration has endorsed it as a replacement for the rabbit test.

Although LAL is favored as a pyrogen test, some parenteral products cannot be tested with LAL because the active ingredient interferes with the outcome. These products must be tested with the rabbit pyrogen test. Such products include:

- meperidine HCl
- promethazine HCl
- oxacillin sodium
- sulfisoxazole
- vancomycin HCl

One strategy to overcome the interference of the active ingredient when using the LAL test is to dilute the product more than two-fold. This allows for some of the aforementioned products to be tested using the LAL test.

CHAPTER HIGHLIGHTS

- Quality assurance programs are in place to monitor, evaluate, correct, and improve the activities and processes in the preparation of sterile products.
- Compounding personnel bear the greatest responsibility in the quality assurance of CSPs.
- Media-fill testing is one method of assessing the aseptic compounding abilities of personnel.
- Garbing, hand washing, and gloved fingertip sampling are annually evaluated for compounding personnel.
- Determining a manner of sterilization depends on the type of product that is being sterilized.
- Physically and visually examining CSPs for contamination can take place immediately after compounding or after the CSP has been stored.

- Positive sterility testing leads to multiple evaluative steps to determine the point in the process at which contamination occurred.
- Pyrogen testing can take different forms depending on the type of product being tested.

QUICK QUIZ

Answer the following multiple-choice questions.

1. Which of the following is a component of a quality assurance program?
   a. a description of monitoring and evaluation activities
   b. the flowchart of personnel in the facility
   c. a list of hazardous CSPs
   d. emergency contact information for the U.S. Food and Drug Administration
2. Compounding personnel must pass hands-on evaluations, including
   a. pyrogen testing
   b. cleaning and disinfecting procedures
   c. hazardous waste disposal
   d. packaging and disbursement procedures
3. Steam sterilization is useful for sterilizing
   a. oils
   b. exposed powders
   c. fats
   d. glassware
4. Visually examining CSPs after preparationis important because
   a. the ingredients might have been incompatible and have precipitated.
   b. the wrong volume may have been injected.
   c. their beyond-use dates may have passed.
   d. they may require refrigeration.
5. The most accurate pyrogen testing is
   a. rabbit testing.
   b. LAL testing.
   c. oxidation testing.
   d. potassium permanganate testing.

Please answer each of the following questions in one to three sentences.

1. Describe at least 5 things that compounding personnel are responsible for ensuring in a compounding facility.

2. Explain why personnel would not wash their gloves in 70% sterile IPA during the gloved fingertip assessment.

3. Name the five types of sterilization, and tell which one is the least utilized and why.

_____

_____

4. Describe the two types of pyrogen testing.

_____

_____

5. Describe what should be done if a high-risk CSP is dispensed but is later found to be contaminated.

_____

_____

Label the following statements as either true or false.

1. ____ Compounding personnel are only required to pass a written testing of their knowledge of aseptic procedures.
2. ____ Personal protective equipment is left on the clean side of the ante-area.
3. ____ Media-fill testing requirements are the same for all CSP risk levels.
4. ____ Filtration is the most commonly used method of sterilization in hospitals.
5. ____ High-risk CSPs are held from distribution until the results of their sterility tests are available.

Match the term in the left column with the correct description from the right column.

1. sterilization
2. quality assurance
3. media-fill test
4. filtration
5. pyrogen

a. passage of a fluid or solution through a sterilizing grade membrane to produce a sterile effluent
b. a test used to qualify the aseptic technique of compounding personnel or processes and to ensure that the processes used produce a sterile product without microbial contamination
c. fever-producing organic substance arising from microbial contamination
d. the destruction of all living organisms and their spores or their complete removal from a preparation
e. the set of activities used to ensure that the procedures used in the preparation of sterile products lead to products that meet predetermined standards of quality.

Answers to Quick Quiz Questions

Chapter 1

Answer the following multiple-choice questions.

1. c.
2. b.
3. d.
4. a.
5. d.

Please answer each of the following questions in a few sentences.

1. Certain compounds are administered where the body's natural defenses can filter or destroy any unwanted substances. For example, inhalants must pass through the respiratory system, which will naturally filter these products before any unwanted particles reach the lungs. Another example is an enteral, which must pass through the stomach. Pyrogens and other contaminants cannot survive the hydrochloric acid produced by the stomach.
2. A central venous catheter line is placed into a large vein in the neck, chest, or groin. It can stay in place for a few days to several months and is used for chemotherapy drugs, long-term antibiotic therapy, or parenteral nutrition solutions. A peripheral catheter line is inserted in either the arms or the hands and is changed every one to three days.
3. Intravenous—injected directly into the vein; subcutaneous—injected into the tissues between the skin and muscle; intramuscular—injected into muscle tissue; intradermal—injected below the upper layer of skin.
4. IV push—a small volume of medicine injected into a vein and administered over a short period of time. Intravenous infusion—administered either continuously or intermittently. Continuous infusion—a volume of 250 mL or more is injected into a vein and administered at a constant flow rate. Intermittent infusion—a volume of 500 mL or less is given over a shorter time period than a continuous infusion and combined with other fluids.
5. (Possible answer) A laminar-airflow workbench is maintained and certified regularly. Detailed cleaning and sanitizing procedures are followed to maintain the cleanliness of the compounding environment.

Answer the following statements as either true or false.

1. False
2. True
3. False
4. False
5. False

Match the term in the left column with the correct description from the right column.

1. c.
2. e.
3. d.
4. a.
5. b.

Chapter 2

Answer the following multiple-choice questions.

1. c.
2. b.
3. a.
4. d.
5. c.

Please answer each of the following questions in one to three sentences.

1. A critical site is a specific place where contaminants may come into contact with a CSP. The tip of a syringe is an example of a critical site. A critical area is a location where CSPs are exposed to possible contamination. A laminar airflow workbench is an example of a critical area.
2. Contaminants are fibers, particles, or microbes that affect the potency and/or stability of a CSP. Fibers from clothing, particles from skin or hair, and microbes such as bacteria, viruses, or fungi are examples of contaminants.
3. Contamination of CSPs can be prevented by following aseptic technique when preparing CSPs. This means proper scrubbing, appropriate garb, and correct handling of CSPs.
4. The pH of the CSP should match the pH of the body area or body part with which it will come into contact. The pH of human blood is about 7.4. The pH of

the CSP should also have a pH of 7.4, or the incompatibility will cause a reaction.
5. The osmolarity of a solution tells you what the concentration of solute is. This is important because osmolarity is a measure of the tonicity of a solution.

Answer the following questions as either true or false.

1. True
2. False
3. False
4. False
5. True

Match the term in the left column with the correct description from the right column.

1. b.
2. a.
3. d.
4. e.
5. c.

Chapter 3

Answer the following multiple-choice questions.

1. a.
2. c.
3. d.
4. d.
5. b.

Please answer each of the following questions in one to three sentences.

1. A loading dose is a dose of medication designed to raise blood levels quickly. The maintenance dose is designed to keep blood levels stable for a longer period of time; it is also known as the daily dose.
2. Osmolarity is measured as the number of particles per liter. Osmolality is measured as the number of particles per kilogram.
3. Alligation is a method for calculating the relative amounts of ingredients of different percentage strengths to use when making up a product of a given strength.
4. $$\frac{1000mL}{20hr} = \frac{XmL}{hr}$$

   50 mL = X
   Flow rate is 50 mL/hr
5. The solution D5W contains 5% dextrose and water. The solution D5 ½NS contains 5% dextrose and 0.45% normal saline.

Label the following statements as either true or false.

1. True
2. False

3. False
4. True
5. False

Match the term in the left column with the correct description from the right column.

1. c
2. e.
3. a.
4. b.
5. d

Chapter 4

Answer the following multiple-choice questions.

1. a.
2. d.
3. d.
4. c.
5. b.

Please answer each of the following questions in one to three sentences.

1. Calibrations are graduated markings on the outside of a syringe barrel measured in increments of 1.0 mL, 0.1 mL, or 0.2 mL. Calibrations are used to measure the volume of fluid in the barrel.
2. The smaller the gauge, the larger the diameter of the opening; the higher the gauge, the smaller the diameter of the opening. The gauge is selected according to the type and volume of fluid being injected or withdrawn. For injections, higher-gauge needles (thinner needles) are more comfortable for the patient.
3. Both are used as CSP containers. Both are made of either glass or plastic. A multiple-dose vial has more than one dose and has preservatives added to its contents. A single-dose vial contains only one dose, and contains no preservatives.
4. A luer-lock syringe uses a needle that screws into the syringe tip. A slip-tip syringe allows the needle to be easily slipped or pressed on. The luer-lock is more efficient in preventing leaks.
5. The large-volume IV delivers fluids to a patient on a continuous basis. It usually contains 500 mL to 1000 mL of fluid. IV piggybacks are small bags of supplements or vitamins that are administered on a set schedule, usually two to three times a day. Piggybacks usually contain 50 mL to 250 mL of solution. They are often attached to large-volume IVs when a patient needs both fluid and the supplemental solution.

Label the following statements as either true or false.

1. False
2. True

3. True
4. False
5. True

Match the term in the left column with the correct description from the right column.

1. c.
2. a.
3. b.
4. e.
5. d.

Chapter 5

Answer the following multiple-choice questions.

1. b.
2. a.
3. c.
4. a.
5. c.

Please answer each of the following questions in one to three sentences.

1. When the surfaces in a clean room are compromised with nicks and cracks, they can harbor harmful microorganisms that can become surface and air contaminants. Some disinfectants can cause damage to surfaces that meet clean room criteria, so it's important that the disinfectants are mild, but still effective.
2. A positive-pressure room is one in which the air pressure is higher than in adjacent spaces, so the air flows out of the room; such as a physically separated room used for high-risk or hazardous compounding activities. A negative-pressure room is one in which the air pressure is lower than in adjacent spaces, so that air flows into the room; this room should be used to contain hazardous materials because of their volatile nature.
3. Activities in an ISO Class 7 area include the preparation of CSPs and the staging of compounding components and supplies. Examples include the clean room, buffer area, and ante-area.
4. Contaminants can easily pass into other areas by being blown, dragged, or trafficked by the movement of personnel when compounding is done out in the open. Traffic flow in and out of the buffer area should be minimized. The segregated compounding area should be away from a high-traffic area. The PEC should be placed out of the flow of personnel traffic. Traffic in the area of the DCA must be controlled.
5. The number of personnel working in the room, the type of compounding processes in use, and temperature effects determine the ACPH value for a work area.

Label the following statements as either true or false.

1. False
2. True
3. True
4. False
5. True

Match the term in the left column with the correct description from the right column.

1. c.
2. a.
3. d.
4. e.
5. b.

Chapter 6

Answer the following multiple-choice questions.

1. d.
2. a.
3. d.
4. b.
5. a.

Please answer each of the following questions in one to three sentences.

1. Possible answer—A hair cover is a soft, disposable low-particulate cap that fits over the head, covering the hair. A face mask is a soft, disposable low-particulate cover worn over the mouth and nose.
2. People who are allergic or sensitive to latex use non-latex gloves.
3. After washing your hands, gently pat them from fingertip to elbow dry using a low-particulate towel or electric dryer.
4. An antimicrobial agent is a soap that washes away bacteria and other pathogens. Antimicrobial agents are used for aseptic hand washing.
5. 1. Take off all jewelry first; 2. Scrub vigorously for 30 seconds; 3. Use an antimicrobial agent.

Label the following statements as either true or false.

1. False
2. False
3. True
4. False
5. False

Match the term in the left column with the correct description from the right column.

1. b.
2. a.
3. e.

4. d.
5. c.

Chapter 7

Answer the following multiple-choice questions.

1. c.
2. d.
3. c.
4. d.
5. b.

Please answer each of the following questions in one to three sentences.

1. (1) Swirling the ampule in an upright motion; (2) Tapping the head of the ampule with a finger; Inverting the ampule and quickly swinging it back into an upright position.
2. Positive pressure occurs when the pressure inside a vial or bottle is greater than the pressure outside of it. This happens when air or liquid is injected into the closed system without removing any air or liquid first. Negative pressure occurs when the pressure outside a vial or bottle is greater than the pressure inside of it. This creates a vacuum effect, making it extremely difficult to withdraw any solution from a vial.
3. Air bubbles take up space that should be occupied by solution. When you're working with extremely small amounts, such as a fraction of a milliliter, any air that is contained within the syringe can greatly affect the amount of drug drawn up. Removing air bubbles results in accurate measurements of solutions.
4. (1) Wipe the rubber top of the vial with alcohol and allow it to dry. (2) Ensure that the needle is firmly attached to the syringe. (3) Pull the plunger back and forth to lubricate the barrel, then pull the plunger back on the syringe to slightly less than the amount of solution you need to draw. (4) Remove the needle cap. Find the center of the stopper on top of the vial, and hold the needle with the bevel end facing up at a 30 degree angle. (5) As you begin to enter the rubber stopper, swing the needle up to a 90 degree angle and fully enter the vial. (6) Invert the vial and needle without shadowing, and slowly push the air from the syringe into the vial. (7) Pull back on the plunger until you withdraw the desired amount from the vial. (8) Remove any air bubbles from the syringe. (You'll learn more about this later in the chapter.) (9) Invert the vial and needle without shadowing, and withdraw the needle and carefully recap the end or inject it into the IV bag injection port and slowly inject.
5. Answer should include 5 of the following: the patient's name or other patient ID (for patient-specific products); control or lot numbers; all solution and ingredient names, amounts, strengths, and concentrations; the total volume; the prescribed administration regimen; expiration date; time (if it's an immediate-use drug); auxiliary labeling; storage requirements (temperature, light-sensitivity, etc.); identification of the responsible pharmacist; device-specific instructions.

Label the following statements as either true or false.

1. True
2. False
3. True
4. False
5. True

Match the term in the left column with the correct description from the right column.

1. c.
2. d.
3. a.
4. e.
5. b.

Chapter 8

Answer the following multiple-choice questions.

1. a.
2. d.
3. c.
4. a.
5. d.

Please answer each of the following questions in one to three sentences.

1. TPNs must be sterile or prepared aseptically to prevent contamination and because the IV administration bypasses the body's natural defenses.
2. PCA stands for patient controlled analgesia. It is used so that patient's can control their own pain medication. This makes it easier to regulate pain.
3. Pediatric patients are smaller and often have undeveloped organs. Therefore, they require a weaker dose than that prescribed for adults.
4. Calcium and phosphorous can form a precipitate if not added in the correct amounts, and in the correct order. The precipitate can block the flow of the TPN.
5. Insulin syringes are calibrated in units instead of mLs.

Answer the following questions as either true or false.

1. False
2. True
3. False
4. False
5. True

Match the term in the left column with the correct description from the right column.

1. e.
2. b.
3. d.
4. a.
5. c.

Chapter 9

Answer the following multiple-choice questions.

1. a.
2. b.
3. d.
4. a.
5. b.

Please answer each of the following questions in one to three sentences.

1. They must ensure that CSPs are accurately identified, measured, diluted, and mixed; CSPs are correctly purified, sterilized, packaged, sealed, labeled, stored, dispensed, and distributed; appropriate cleanliness conditions are being maintained; labeling and supplementary instructions are provided for the proper clinical administration of CSPs
2. Rinsing their gloves would remove any microorganisms or contaminants from their gloves, which would result in a false-negative outcome. Since the gloved-fingertip test is assessing whether sterile steps are being taken during garbing, this would negate the results.
3. The five types of sterilization are dry heat, steam, filtration, gas, and ionizing radiation. Ionizing radiation is the least used because it is cost-prohibitive and the radiation can affect the product or the container in which the product is being stored.
4. **Rabbit testing:** (1) Selecting three rabbits, then render the syringes, glassware, and needles free from pyrogens by heating at 250°C for no less than 30 minutes or by another suitable method; (2) warm the product to be tested to $37 \pm 2°C$; (3) Into an ear vein in each of three rabbits, inject 10 mL of the product per kilogram of body weight, completing each injecting within 10 minutes of the start of administration; (4) Record the rabbit body temperatures at 30-minute intervals 1 to 3 hours after the injection; If no rabbit shows an individual increase in temperature of 0.5°C or more, the product meets the requirement for the absence of pyrogens. If any rabbit shows and individual temperature increase of 0.5°C or more, continue the test using five other rabbits. If not more than three of the eight rabbits show individual increases of 0.5°C or more, and if the sum of the eight individual maximal temperature increases does not exceed 3.3°C, the material under examination meets the requirements for the absence of pyrogens.

    LSL procedure: The *Limulus* amebocyte lysate test requires the use of an extract from the blood cells of the horseshoe crab, which contains an enzyme and protein system that coagulates in the presence of low levels of lipopolysaccharides.
5. The documentation should be pulled for the testing of the CSP; the location of the suspected contaminated products should be determined; the physician of the patient who received the product should be contacted and informed of the possible contamination risks involving the product.

Label the following statements as either true or false.

1. False
2. True
3. False
4. True
5. False

Match the term in the left column with the correct description from the right column.

1. d.
2. e.
3. b.
4. a.
5. c.

Abbreviations Commonly Used in Prescriptions and Medication Orders

Abbreviation	Meaning
a	before
ac	before meals
am	before noon
ad	right ear
as	left ear
au	both ears
bid	twice a day
d	day
gtt	drops
h	hour
hs	at hour of sleep (bedtime)
noc	night
od	right eye
os	left eye
ou	both eyes
p	after
pc	after meals
pm	after noon
po	oral or by mouth
pr	per rectum
prn	as needed
q	every
qd	every day
qh	every hour
qod	every other day
q2h	every 2 hours
qid	four times a day
ss	one-half
stat	immediately
supp	suppository
tid	three times a day
tiw	three times a week
wk	week
yr	year

Nomograms for Determination of Body Surface Area from Height and Weight

Nomogram for Determination of Body Surface Area From Height and Weight

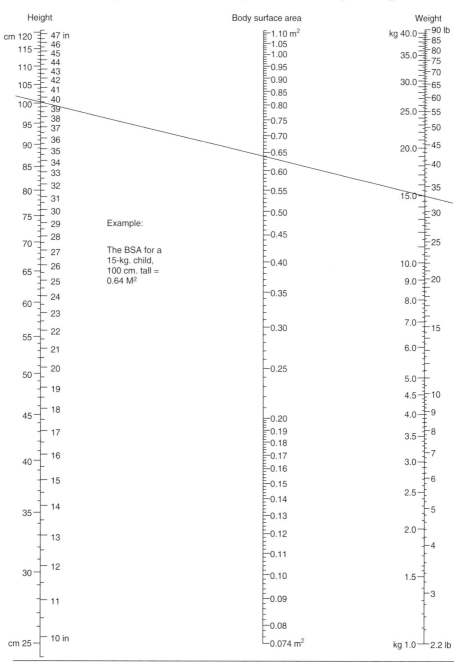

Example:

The BSA for a 15-kg. child, 100 cm. tall = 0.64 M^2

From the formula of Du Bots and Du Bots, *Arch. intern. Med.*, 17, 863 (1916): $S = W^{0.425} \times H^{0.725} \times 71.84$, or log S = log $W \times 0.425$ + log $H \times 0.725$ + 1.8564 (S = body surface in cm^2, W = weight in kg, H = height in cm).

Nomogram for Determination of Body Surface Area From Height and Weight

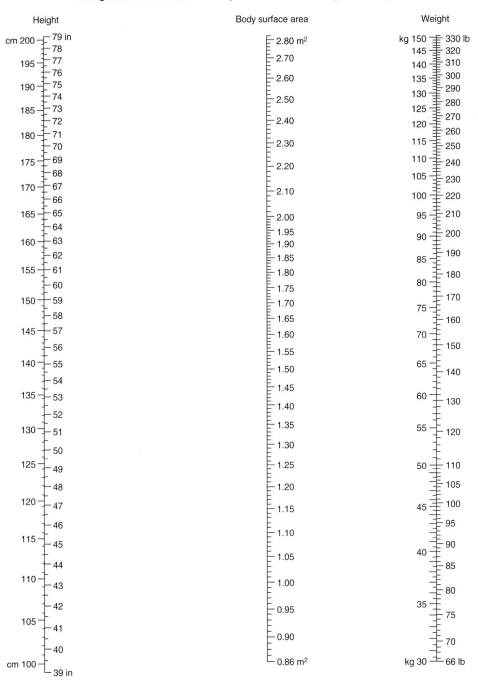

From the formula of Du Bots and Du Bots, *Arch. intern. Med.*, 17, 863 (1916): $S = W^{0.425} \times H^{0.725} \times 71.84$, or log S = log $W \times 0.425$ + log $H \times 0.725$ + 1.8564 (S = body surface in cm², W = weight in kg, H = height in cm).

Body Mass Index Charts

Normal, Overweight, and Obese Body Mass Index

BMI	Normal						Overweight					Obese									
	19	20	21	22	23	24	25	26	27	28	29	30	31	32	33	34	35	36	37	38	39
Height (inches)											Body Weight (pounds)										
58	91	96	100	105	110	115	119	124	129	134	138	143	148	153	158	162	167	172	177	181	186
59	94	99	104	109	114	119	124	128	133	138	143	148	15	158	163	168	173	178	183	188	193
60	97	102	107	112	118	123	128	133	138	143	148	153	158	163	168	174	179	184	189	194	199
61	100	106	111	116	122	127	132	137	143	148	153	158	164	169	174	180	185	190	195	201	206
62	104	109	115	120	126	131	136	142	147	153	158	164	169	175	180	186	191	196	202	207	213
63	107	113	118	124	130	135	141	146	152	158	163	169	175	180	186	191	197	203	208	214	220
64	110	116	122	128	134	140	145	151	157	163	169	174	180	186	192	197	204	209	215	221	227
65	114	120	126	132	138	144	150	156	162	178	174	180	186	192	198	204	210	216	222	228	234
66	118	124	130	136	142	148	155	161	167	173	179	186	192	198	204	210	216	223	229	235	241
67	121	127	134	140	146	153	159	166	172	178	185	191	198	204	211	217	223	230	236	242	249
68	125	131	138	144	151	158	164	171	177	184	190	197	203	210	216	223	230	236	243	249	256
69	128	135	142	149	155	162	169	176	182	189	196	203	209	216	223	230	236	243	250	257	263
70	132	139	146	153	160	167	174	181	188	195	202	209	216	222	229	236	243	250	257	264	271
71	136	143	150	157	165	172	179	186	193	200	208	215	222	229	236	243	250	257	265	272	279
72	140	147	154	162	169	177	184	191	199	206	213	221	228	235	242	250	258	265	272	279	287
73	144	151	159	166	174	182	189	197	204	212	219	227	235	242	250	257	265	272	280	288	295
74	148	155	163	171	179	186	194	202	210	218	225	233	241	249	256	264	272	280	287	295	303
75	152	160	168	176	184	192	200	208	216	224	232	240	248	256	264	272	279	287	295	303	311
76	156	164	172	180	189	197	205	213	221	230	238	246	254	263	271	279	287	295	304	312	320

Extremely Obese Body Mass Index

Extremely Obese

BMI	40	41	42	43	44	45	46	47	48	49	50	51	52	53	54
Height (inches)							Body Weight (pounds)								
58	191	196	201	205	210	215	220	224	229	234	239	244	248	253	258
59	198	203	208	212	217	222	227	232	237	242	247	252	257	262	267
60	204	209	215	220	225	230	235	240	245	250	255	261	266	271	276
61	211	217	222	227	232	238	243	248	254	259	264	269	275	280	285
62	218	224	229	235	240	246	251	256	262	267	273	278	284	289	295
63	225	231	237	242	248	254	259	265	270	278	282	287	293	299	304
64	232	238	244	250	256	262	267	273	279	285	291	296	302	308	314
65	240	246	252	258	264	270	276	282	288	294	300	306	312	318	324
66	247	253	260	266	272	278	284	291	297	303	309	315	322	328	334
67	255	261	268	274	280	287	293	299	306	312	319	325	331	338	344
68	262	269	276	282	289	295	302	308	315	322	328	335	341	348	354
69	270	277	284	291	297	304	311	318	324	331	338	345	351	358	365
70	278	285	292	299	306	313	320	327	334	341	348	355	362	369	376
71	286	293	301	308	315	322	329	338	343	351	358	365	372	379	386
72	294	302	309	316	324	331	338	346	353	361	368	375	383	390	397
73	302	310	318	325	333	340	348	355	363	371	378	386	393	401	408
74	311	319	326	334	342	350	358	365	373	381	389	396	404	412	420
75	319	327	335	343	351	359	367	375	383	391	399	407	415	423	431
76	328	336	344	353	361	369	377	385	394	402	410	418	426	435	443

Pediatric Body Mass Index

Calculated Body Mass Index

29"- 43" and 35 lbs.- 43 lbs.

Whenever a child's specific height and weight measurement are not included, refer to the closest number in the table.

Weight header — top value = **Kg**, second row = **Lb**. Left columns = Height (**Cm** / **In**).

Height Cm	In	15.9	16.1	16.3	16.6	16.8	17.0	17.2	17.5	17.7	17.9	18.1	18.4	18.6	18.8	19.1	19.3	19.5
Lb		35	35.5	36	36.5	37	37.5	38	38.5	39	39.5	40	40.5	41	41.5	42	42.5	43
73.7	29	29.3	29.7	30.1	30.4	30.9	31.3	31.8	32.2	32.6	33.0	33.4	33.9	34.3	34.7			
74.9	29.5	28.3	28.7	29.1	29.5	29.9	30.3	30.7	31.1	31.5	31.9	32.3	32.7	33.1	33.5	33.9	34.3	34.7
76.2	30	27.3	27.7	28.1	28.5	28.9	29.3	29.7	30.1	30.5	30.9	31.2	31.6	32.0	32.4	32.8	33.2	33.6
77.5	30.5	26.5	26.8	27.2	27.6	28.0	28.3	28.7	29.1	29.5	29.9	30.2	30.6	31.0	31.4	31.7	32.1	32.5
78.7	31	25.6	26.0	26.3	26.7	27.1	27.4	27.8	28.2	28.5	28.9	29.3	29.6	30.0	30.4	30.7	31.1	31.5
80.0	31.5	24.8	25.2	25.5	25.9	26.2	26.6	26.9	27.3	27.6	28.0	28.3	28.7	29.1	29.4	29.8	30.1	30.5
81.3	32	24.0	24.4	24.7	25.1	25.4	25.7	26.1	26.4	26.8	27.1	27.5	27.8	28.2	28.5	28.8	29.2	29.5
82.6	32.5	23.3	23.6	24.0	24.3	24.6	25.0	25.3	25.6	26.0	26.3	26.6	27.0	27.3	27.6	28.0	28.3	28.5
83.8	33	22.6	22.9	23.2	23.6	23.9	24.2	24.5	24.9	25.2	25.5	25.8	26.1	26.5	26.8	27.1	27.4	27.8
85.1	33.5	21.9	22.2	22.6	22.9	23.2	23.5	23.8	24.1	24.4	24.7	25.1	25.4	25.7	26.0	26.3	26.6	26.9
86.4	34	21.3	21.6	21.9	22.2	22.5	22.8	23.1	23.4	23.7	24.0	24.3	24.6	24.9	25.2	25.5	25.8	26.2
87.6	34.5	20.7	21.0	21.3	21.6	21.9	22.2	22.4	22.7	23.0	23.3	23.6	23.9	24.2	24.5	24.8	25.1	25.4
88.9	35	20.1	20.4	20.7	20.9	21.2	21.5	21.8	22.1	22.4	22.7	23.0	23.2	23.5	23.8	24.1	24.4	24.7
90.2	35.5	19.5	19.8	20.1	20.4	20.6	20.9	21.2	21.5	21.8	22.0	22.3	22.6	22.9	23.2	23.4	23.7	24.0
91.4	36	19.0	19.3	19.5	19.8	20.1	20.3	20.6	20.9	21.2	21.4	21.7	22.0	22.2	22.5	22.8	23.1	23.3
92.7	36.5	18.5	18.7	19.0	19.3	19.5	19.8	20.1	20.3	20.6	20.8	21.1	21.4	21.6	21.9	22.2	22.4	22.7
94.0	37	18.0	18.2	18.5	18.7	19.0	19.3	19.5	19.8	20.0	20.3	20.5	20.8	21.1	21.3	21.6	21.8	22.1
95.3	37.5	17.5	17.7	18.0	18.2	18.5	18.7	19.0	19.2	19.5	19.7	20.0	20.2	20.5	20.7	21.0	21.2	21.5
96.5	38	17.0	17.3	17.5	17.8	18.0	18.3	18.5	18.7	19.0	19.2	19.5	19.7	20.0	20.2	20.4	20.7	20.9
97.8	38.5	16.6	16.8	17.1	17.3	17.6	17.8	18.0	18.3	18.5	18.7	19.0	19.2	19.4	19.7	19.9	20.2	20.4
99.1	39	16.2	16.4	16.6	16.9	17.1	17.3	17.6	17.8	18.0	18.3	18.5	18.7	19.0	19.2	19.4	19.6	19.9
100.3	39.5	15.8	16.0	16.2	16.4	16.7	16.9	17.1	17.3	17.6	17.8	18.0	18.2	18.5	18.7	18.9	19.2	19.4
101.6	40	15.4	15.6	15.8	16.0	16.3	16.5	16.7	16.9	17.1	17.4	17.6	17.8	18.0	18.2	18.5	18.7	18.9
102.9	40.5	15.0	15.2	15.4	15.6	15.9	16.1	16.3	16.5	16.7	16.9	17.1	17.4	17.6	17.8	18.0	18.2	18.4
104.1	41	14.6	14.8	15.1	15.3	15.5	15.7	15.9	16.1	16.3	16.5	16.7	16.9	17.1	17.4	17.6	17.8	18.0
105.4	41.5	14.3	14.5	14.7	14.9	15.1	15.3	15.5	15.7	15.9	16.1	16.3	16.5	16.7	16.9	17.1	17.3	17.6
106.7	42	13.9	14.1	14.3	14.5	14.7	14.9	15.1	15.3	15.5	15.7	15.9	16.1	16.3	16.5	16.7	16.9	17.1
108.0	42.5	13.6	13.8	14.0	14.2	14.4	14.6	14.8	15.0	15.2	15.4	15.6	15.8	16.0	16.2	16.3	16.5	16.7
109.2	43	13.3	13.5	13.7	13.9	14.1	14.3	14.4	14.6	14.8	15.0	15.2	15.4	15.6	15.8	16.0	16.2	16.4

Equivalency Tables

Equivalences of Common Metric Measurements

1,000 mm	100 cm
100 cm	1 m
1,000 mL	1 L
10 cc	1 mL
1,000 mcg	1 mg
1,000 mg	1 g
1,000 g	1 kg

Common Household Abbreviations and Equivalents

Abbreviation	Unit	Equivalent
gtt	Drop	n/a
tsp	Teaspoon	n/a
tbs	Tablespoon	1 tbs = 3 tsp
oz	Fluidounce	2 tbs = 1 oz
oz	Ounce (weight)	16 oz = 1 lb
cup	Cup	1 cup = 8 oz
pt	Pint	1 pint = 2 cups
qt	Quart	1 quart = 4 cups = 2 pt

Apothecaries' System Basics

Liquid Volume

60 minims (m)	1 fluidram
8 fluidrams	1 fluid ounce (oz)
16 fluid oz	1 pint (pt)
2 pt	1 quart (qt)

Solid Weight

60 grains (gr)	1 dram
8 drams	1 oz
12 oz	1 pound (lb)

Conversion Equivalents of Volume

Apothecary Measure	Approximate Metric Equivalent (mL)	Exact Metric Equivalent (mL)
1 fl oz	30	29.57
4 fl oz	120	118.28
1 pt (16 fl oz)a	480	473.00
1 qt (2 pt)	960	946.00
1 gal (4 qt)	3,840	3,785.00

Conversion Equivalents of Weight

Apothecary or Avoirdupois Measure	Approximate Metric Equivalent	Exact Metric Equivalent
1 avoir oz	30 g	28.35 g
1 avoir lb (16 oz)		454 g
2.2 avoir lb	1 kg	1,000 g

Common Household Measures

Household Measure	Approximate Equivalent	Apothecary Equivalent	Other Equivalent
½ tsp	2.5 mL	n/a	n/a
1 tsp	5 mL	1 fluidram	n/a
3 tsp	15 mL	n/a	1 tbs or ½ oz
2 tbs	30 mL	1 fl oz	1 oz

Glossary

Absorption—the process that occurs when an ingredient is soaked up by the CSP container and results in loss of drug

ABW—actual body weight

ACPH—air changes per hour

active ingredient—the substance or chemical responsible for the action of the finished product

adsorption—the process that occurs when an ingredient adheres to the surface of the CSP container and results in loss of drug

agar—a gelatinous substance used to collect cultures

allergen extract—a biologic that is used to test for an allergy

alligation—the calculation of the relative amount of ingredients of different percentage strengths to make up a product of a given strength

ampule—a sealed glass container that contains a single dose of medication

ante-area—the vicinity located directly outside the clean room; the first line of air-quality control in a clean room layout

ante room—a room located directly outside the clean room where gowning occurs and compounding supplies are stored

antimicrobial soap—an agent that kills microscopic pathogens such as bacteria and other potentially harmful organisms

antineoplastic—a chemical that slows down or prevents the growth and reproduction of cancerous cells

autoclave—a machine invented in 1879 to sterilize equipment and other objects using superheated water and pressurized steam

B

bevel—the slanted, pointed tip of a needle

beyond-use date—the date after which a product must not be used; determined by the pharmacist from the date and time the product is prepared

biologic—a substance produced by a living source

biologic indicator—a special preparation of microorganisms that are known to be resistant to a particular sterilization process

biological safety cabinet (BSC)—a vertical flow hood that uses HEPA-filtered air that flows vertically (from the top of the hood towards the work surface) to provide an aseptic work area

BSA—body surface area

buffer—a compound or mixture of compounds that helps prevent changes in pH

buffer area—the vicinity where the PEC is located and where CSP supplies are prepared

C

calibrations—graduated markings on the outside of a syringe barrel

catheter—a tiny delivery or drainage tube that is inserted into a vein, artery, or body cavity

chemo mat—a special device placed outside the BSC to absorb any leaks or spills

chemotherapy—the use of chemicals to treat a disease, especially cancer

chlorohexidene gluconate—an antimicrobial soap used for aseptic hand washing, often abbreviated CHG

clean room—a room in which the air quality, temperature, and humidity are highly regulated to reduce the risk of cross-contamination

closed-system containers—receptacles in which air cannot flow freely in or out

closed system transfer device (CSTD)—a special system for transferring hazardous drugs from one container to another

cold chain—the steps taken to keep a biologic at a specific low temperature from the manufacturer's refrigerator to the pharmacy, clinic, or doctor's office where it is administered'

compatibility—a property that describes how effectively one product will combine with another product

compounded sterile product (CSP)—a mixture of one or more substances that is made free of contamination before use

compounding aseptic containment isolator (CACI)—a CAI that is designed to protect the worker as well as the product; used to compound hazardous drugs

contaminant—any unwanted particulate matter or fever-inducing agent

continuous infusion—when a volume of 250 mL or more is injected into a vein and administered at a constant flow rate

coring—transferring a part of the rubber stopper of a vial or container into a solution because of improper needle stick

Corynebacterium—bacteria found on the skin's surface

critical area—an ISO Class 5 environment in which CSPs are prepared (e.g., laminar airflow workbench, biological safety cabinet)

critical site—any location where contaminants might come into contact with a CSP; these locations are either never touched (e.g., needle, needle hub, syringe plunger) or swabbed with alcohol prior to needle entry (e.g., ampule, vial stopper)

critical surface—any surface that comes into contact with a sterile product, container, or closure

cytotoxic—a chemical that poisons cells so that they are not able to reproduce or grow

D

D5W—dextrose 5% in water; commonly used base solution for CSPs

daily dose—the amount of a drug to be taken over 24 hours

delivery system—the pieces of equipment that allow a drug to follow a designated route of administration into the body

diabetes mellitus—disease which results when a person's body does not produce enough insulin

diluent—a product that is added to a solution to reduce its strength, or dilute it

dilution—a process that makes a more concentrated substance less concentrated

dimensional analysis—a problem-solving method in which any number or expression can be multiplied by one without changing its value

direct compounding area (DCA)—a critical area in the primary engineering control in which critical sites are exposed to unidirectional HEPA-filtered air

E

endotoxins—compounds found inside infectious agents such as bacteria

essential amino acids—amino acids which are not produced by the body and must therefore be supplied through the diet

expiration date—the date after which a product must not be used; determined by the manufacturer for an unopened and properly stored product

F

filter needle—a needle with a filter molded into the hub designed for one-time use only; used to remove glass particles from a solution

filter straws—thin, sterile straws with a filter molded into the hub; used to draw fluid from an ampule

filtration—the passage of a fluid or solution through a sterilizing grade membrane to produce a sterile effluent

G

garb—all elements of personal protective equipment

gauge—the diameter of the opening of a needle, or the lumen

H

hazardous drug—a drug that can cause serious effects such as cancer, organ toxicity, fertility problems, genetic damage, or birth defects

hemodialysis—type of dialysis used to remove toxic substances from the blood

HEPA filter—a high-efficiency particulate air filter used in all aseptic processing areas

hypodermic needle—a needle that fits on the end of a syringe used to inject fluids into or withdraw fluids out of the body

I

IBW—ideal body weight

incompatibility—a property that describes the negative effect of combining one sterile product with another sterile product, surface, or material

infusion pump—an automatic device used with an IV system for delivering medication at regular intervals in specific quantities

IPA—isopropyl alcohol

insulin pump—lightweight pump that maintains blood glucose levels at a normal level

intermittent infusion—when a volume of 500 mL or less is given over a shorter time period than a continuous infusion and combined with other fluids

intravenous (IV) admixture—a CSP in which a measured substance is added to a 50 mL or larger bag or bottle of IV fluid

intravenous piggybacks (IVPBs)—IV bags that are administered on a set schedule

intravenous push (IVP)—a method of drug administration in which a small volume of medicine (less than 250 mL) is injected into a vein and administered over a short period of time

isotonic solution—a solution with an osmotic pressure equal to that of the inside of a body cell

L

laminar airflow workbench (LAFW)—a workbench that uses HEPA-filtered air that flows horizontally (from the back of the bench towards you) to provide an aseptic work area

laminar flow—air flow that moves in parallel from ceiling to floor or from wall to wall with uniform velocity and minimal turbulence

LBW—lean body weight

loading dose—a large initial dose required to achieve the desired blood drug level given at the beginning of a therapeutic regimen

lumen—the hollow part of a needle

M

maintenance dose—a smaller dose following the loading dose to sustain the desired drug blood level or drug effect

malignant—cancerous

media-fill test—a test used to qualify the aseptic technique of compounding personnel or processes, and to ensure that the processes used produce a sterile product that is without microbial contamination

microbial contamination—a situation in which microbes such as bacteria, viruses, molds, or yeasts, come into contact with a CSP

N

narrow therapeutic index (NTI)—small room for error.

negative pressure—a condition that occurs when the pressure outside a vial or bottle is greater than the pressure inside of it

negative-pressure room—an area in which the air pressure is lower than in nearby spaces so that air flows into the room

nomogram—a chart that uses the patient's height and weight to estimate the body surface area in square meters

normal saline (NS)—an isotonic solution containing 0.9% sodium chloride; commonly used base solution for CSPs

O

open-system container—a receptacle in which air can pass freely in and out

ophthalmics—drugs applied to the eye

osmolality—the number of osmoles of solute per kilogram of solvent (mOsm/kg)

osmolarity—the number of osmoles of solute per liter of solution (mOsm/L)

otics—drugs applied to the ear

P

parenteral—a compound that is given by injection

peritoneal dialysis—type of dialysis in which a solution is allowed to flow into the peritoneal, or abdominal, cavity in order to remove toxic substances

personnel protective equipment (PPE)—the various pieces of clothing and gear worn by pharmacy technicians to lower the risk of personal infection and the spread of contamination

pH—the measurement of a substance describing how acidic or basic it is

PhaSeal—a type of CSTD that keeps human exposure to chemotherapy drugs to a minimum

positive pressure—a condition that occurs when the pressure inside a vial or bottle is greater than the pressure outside of it

positive-pressure room—an area in which the air pressure is higher than the air pressure in nearby vicinities so that the air flows out of the room

powder volume—the volume that a powder occupies after it is dissolved in a solution

precipitate—a solid formed from a solution or suspension when incompatible ingredients are combined

primary engineering control (PEC)—the equipment that provides an ISO Class 5 environment for the exposure of critical sites when compounding sterile preparations; LAFW, BSC, CAI

product—a commercially manufactured sterile drug that has been evaluated for safety and efficacy by the U.S. Food and Drug Administration

pyrogens—fever-producing organic substances such as bacteria, viruses, or fungi

Q

quality assurance—the set of activities used to ensure that the procedures used in the preparation of sterile products lead to products that meet predetermined standards of quality

R

radiopharmaceutical—a radioactive CSP used in nuclear medicine to diagnose and treat certain diseases

reconstitution—the process in which a diluent is added to a powered form of a drug

rhinitis—the irritation and inflammation of the internal areas of the nose

risk level—the potential threat to patients caused by the introduction of microbial contamination into a finished sterile product

route of administration—the specific way a parenteral or other drug comes into contact with body tissue

S

scrubs—short-sleeved, full-legged, low-particulate garments that can be sterilized and worn under a gown

shadowing—a situation in which the HEPA-filtered airflow in the critical area (BSC) is blocked before reaching the critical site

stability—the ability of the CSP to remain effective until used, or until the expiration date or beyond-use date has been reached

Staphylococcus—bacteria found on the skin's surface or the mouth, nose, or throat; transmitted by direct contact

Sterilization—the destruction of all living organisms and their spores, or their complete removal from a preparation

storage—the area where the CSPs are stored and the container in which each CSP is stored

T

technetium-99m (Tc-99m)—isotope commonly used for compounding radiopharmaceuticals

terminally sterilize—a process used to produce sterility in a final product contained in it's final packaging system

tonicity—a measurement of the way cells and tissues react to a solution that surrounds them

touch contamination—a situation that occurs when physical contact between a CSP and another object results in contamination; this is the most common cause of contamination when preparing CSPs

transfer needles—syringes that have needles on both ends

V

vaccination—the use of a biologic product, a vaccine, to produce active immunity in a patient

vented needle—a needle with side openings used to reconstitute powdered medication

viaflex bags— plastic, sterile IV containers that are not open to contaminants

viscosity—how the fluid is able to flow

W

w/v—weight/volume

Index

Page numbers in *italics* denote figures; those followed by a "t" denote tables.